PARAMEDIC CERTIFICATION EXAM

Sixth Edition

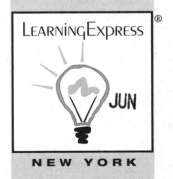

LEARNINGEXPRESS®

JUN

2017

NEW YORK

Cataloging-in-Publication Data is on file with the Library of Congress.

ISBN 978-1-61103-080-8

Printed in the United States of America

9 8 7 6 5 4 3 2 1

Sixth Edition

For more information on LearningExpress, other LearningExpress products, or bulk sales, please write to us at:
224 W. 29th Street
3rd Floor
New York, NY 10001

LIST OF CONTRIBUTORS ▶

Catherine Parvensky Barwell, MEd, RN, PHRN, EMT-I, began as a certified EMT and an EMT instructor. She then obtained her license as a registered nurse (RN) and after practicing for a number of years, returned to emergency medical care as an Emergency Medical Services (EMS) Training Coordinator. She was appointed to a long-term position as County Deputy Director of Training for the Department of Emergency Services where she oversaw all EMS and fire service training as well as public safety education.

Virginia Brennan, PhD, is a linguist and editor in Nashville, Tennessee.

Angel Clark Burba, MS, EMT-P, is an Assistant Professor and Program Coordinator for the paramedic program at Howard Community College in Maryland. She serves on the Education Committee of the National Association of EMS Educators (NAEMSE).

Jan Gallagher, PhD, is an editor living and working in New Jersey.

Bill Garcia, EMT-P, is a founding editor of *Rescue* magazine and serves in the United States Navy. He is based in Maryland.

Dawn S. Pecora, MS, PA, EMT-P, is a part-time faculty member of EMS at the University of Maryland–Baltimore County and a full-time physician assistant. She has been in EMS for 23 years and is a retired lieutenant of the Baltimore County Fire Department.

Elaine Silverstein is a writer and editor living and working in New Jersey.

Steven C. Wood is the EMS coordinator in charge of operations for the county of San Diego, Division of EMS. He has been in EMS for 18 years.

Mike Clumpner, PhD(c), MBA, NREMT-P, CCEMT-P, PNCCT, EMT-T, FP-C, has been a paramedic for 18 years, the last nine years as a helicopter flight paramedic. He is a full-time fire captain with the Charlotte (NC) Fire Department and faculty at the University of Maryland–Baltimore County, University of North Las Vegas, and Harvard University. He has 10 published textbooks and lectured at more than 250 conferences on four continents.

Greg Sharpe, MPA, EMT-P, has been a paramedic for 14 years and has been in EMS for 27 years. He is a full-time battalion chief with the Charlotte (NC) Fire Department and is a regular EMS instructor for the Charlotte (NC) Fire Training Academy. He has several EMT and paramedic exam preparation books published.

CONTENTS

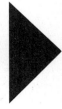

CONTENTS

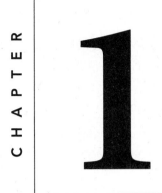

ABOUT THE PARAMEDIC EXAM

CHAPTER SUMMARY

This chapter tells you how to become certified as a Paramedic or NRP. It outlines the certification requirements of the National Registry of Emergency Medical Technicians (NREMT) and tells you how to use this book to study for the written exam.

The National Registry of Emergency Medical Technicians (NREMT) was established in 1970 in response to a suggestion by the U.S. Committee on Highway Safety. Today, the NREMT is an independent nonprofit agency whose job is to certify that EMTs and paramedics have the knowledge and skills to do their jobs—to save lives and preserve health. By setting uniform national standards for training, testing, and continuing education, the NREMT helps ensure patient safety throughout the United States.

In all 50 states, the NREMT and state offices of Emergency Medical Services work together to establish certification requirements for EMTs and paramedics. All states test individuals seeking to become EMTs or paramedics. Some states make sole use of NREMT exams, while others offer state tests. (A list of specific certification requirements for all 50 states appears in Chapter 9.)

IMPORTANT ADDRESS AND PHONE NUMBER

National Registry of Emergency Medical
  Technicians
Rocco V. Morando Building
6610 Busch Boulevard
P.O. Box 29233
Columbus, OH 43229
Telephone: 614-888-4484
Fax: 614-888-8920
www.nremt.org

The curriculum for paramedic education and testing comes from the National Emergency Medical Service Education Standards. The standards were phased in as the basis for educational programs and testing. The NREMT exams and the state tests are all based on these standards. The practice tests in this book and the review of the practical exam in Chapter 8 are also based on these standards. By preparing with this book as a supplement to your paramedic education program, you will be ready to succeed on the paramedic certification exam.

Minimum Certification Requirements

To become certified as a nationally registered Paramedic, an individual must meet the following requirements:

- Be at least 18 years old
- Hold current NREMT or state certification at the Emergency Responder, Emergency Medical Technician, Advanced Emergency Medical Technician, or Paramedic levels
- Successfully complete a state-approved paramedic program that reaches or exceeds the behavioral objectives of the National Emergency Medical Service Education Standards

- Truthfully complete the "Licensing Action and Felony Statement" on the NREMT application and provide documentation required for any positive criminal history
- Possess current CPR for the healthcare provider certification
- Successfully complete the NREMT-Paramedic/ Paramedic cognitive and psychomotor examinations

*If the applicant's initial paramedic training was completed more than two years prior and the individual has maintained state certification at the paramedic level, the individual must submit documentation verifying completion of a paramedic refresher course within the past two years.

If the applicant's initial paramedic training was completed more than two years ago and the individual has never obtained state or NREMT certification, the individual must complete another state-approved paramedic training program in its entirety.

If the individual's initial paramedic training was previously certified by NREMT or a state agency, reentry into the National Registry may be granted provided the individual:

- Submits official documentation of successful completion of DOT paramedic training after January 1, 1977
- Shows satisfactory evidence of prior state certification as a paramedic
- Has current status as an American Heart Association Advanced Cardiac Life Support (ACLS) provider or instructor
- Completed either Prehospital Trauma Life Support (PHTLS) or International Trauma Life Support (ITLS) within the past two years
- Completed a state-approved DOT paramedic refresher training program or 48 hours of advanced life support (ALS) training similar to that of the DOT paramedic refresher training program
- Has a letter of approval from the state EMS office in the state where the individual works or intends to work, supporting such recertification
- Successfully completes the NREMT-Paramedic/Paramedic cognitive and psychomotor examinations

Paramedic certification (now abbreviated as NRP [Nationally Registered Paramedic] by the NREMT) requires successful completion of both cognitive (knowledge-based) and psychomotor (practical skills–based) exams. Successful completion of each exam remains valid for a period of 12 months. If you fail to successfully complete the remaining portion within that 12-month period, you will be required to repeat the original exam. For example, if you pass the cognitive exam but fail one of the stations in the practical exam, you will have 12 months to pass the practical exam or you will be required to retake the cognitive exam. Successful completion of both the practical and cognitive examinations must occur within two years of the completion of a state-approved paramedic training program.

How to Apply

Once you have met all of the requirements previously outlined and are ready to take the certification exams, go to the NREMT website at www.nremt.org to obtain an application and find testing locations. Once you create and access an online account, you will be able to apply online for the certification exams and track your certification progress.

Once the NREMT has confirmed your eligibility, someone will inform you how and where to arrange to take the certification exams. Do not delay making contact with the NREMT, as it is the source of significant useful information on the certification process.

The Paramedic Cognitive Exam

The Paramedic exam uses computer-adaptive testing (CAT). With CAT, each exam is tailored specifically for each candidate. Exams begin with an easy question. If you answer that question correctly, the next question will be slightly more challenging. If the question is answered incorrectly, the next question will be slightly easier. With each correct answer, the computer algorithm statistically estimates your competence. As the exam progresses, the estimation of competence becomes more precise.

Once the CAT algorithm is confident that you have proven competence, it will terminate the exam. This generally occurs after 80 to 110 questions, but may take as many as 150 questions. Based on the way the CAT cognitive exam works, no two exams are exactly the same, although the test question bank from which the computer draws is the same for all exams. The paramedic candidate is allowed two and a half hours to complete the examination. Based on research findings of the actual practice of paramedics nationwide, NREMT developed an examination plan that determined the breakdown of questions for the CAT cognitive examinations. While specific test question selection will be different for each candidate with varying difficulty, the percentage of the exam from each topic area will be the same (see Table 1.1).

TABLE 1.1 BREAKDOWN OF QUESTIONS ON THE EXAMS IN THIS BOOK	
TEST TOPIC	PERCENTAGE OF OVERALL TEST
Airway, Respiration, and Ventilation	17–21%
Cardiology and Resuscitation	17–21%
Patient Assessment–Trauma	18–22%
Medical/Obstetrics/Gynecology	26–30%
EMS Operations	12–16%

In addition to validated test questions, exams also include pilot test questions that have been written but not yet validated. These questions are being evaluated for possible inclusion in future examinations. It is impossible to identify which questions are validated and which are pilot questions, so answer each question to the best of your ability. Pilot questions are not counted toward your exam results.

Exam questions appear on the computer screen one question at a time. Once you provide an answer, the next question will appear. You are not able to go back and change an answer or to mark an answer to revisit later. Therefore, take your time to adequately read and analyze each exam question. Do not rush through your answers. If you do not know the answer, take your best guess and move on.

Whereas the old written certification examination contained 180 questions, requiring 75% accuracy to pass, there is no minimum number of test questions or minimum percentage of correct answers needed to pass the cognitive exam. Rather, the CAT algorithm decides when and if the candidate has demonstrated competency based on the questions answered.

Based on your answers, the computer will determine whether or not you have demonstrated competency and will terminate the exam session. If your answers demonstrate competency, you have passed the exam. Typically, both strong and weak candidates will finish after answering fewer questions than those near entry-level competency.

You will not know when you leave the examination site whether you have passed or failed the exam. Since the exam is tailored to challenge each individual candidate to the limit of his or her ability, everyone taking the exam will think it is difficult. You will be able to find your results through the NREMT's secure website within a couple of days. If you fail the exam, you will be provided information detailing areas in which you need improvement.

Candidates are given three opportunities to pass the cognitive exam provided other criteria for NREMT certification are met. After three unsuccessful attempts, the candidate must complete a 48-hour remedial training program. Following completion of remedial training, the candidate is given three additional attempts to successfully complete the exam. This must all occur within two years of completing the initial paramedic training program. Candidates who fail to pass after a total of six attempts or within the two-year time limit are required to repeat the state-approved paramedic training program in its entirety prior to being able to retake the certification exams.

Candidates who successfully complete the examination will be sent NREMT certification materials. Candidates who fail the exam will receive notification from the NREMT that identifies the areas in which their performance was near or below the passing standard. Their course of study should focus on these identified areas of weakness.

For additional information on the specifics surrounding the certification process, how the CAT was developed, and how certification works, visit the NREMT website at www.nremt.org.

A Word about the CAT Environment

Registered Pearson VUE testing centers administer all CAT exams. You will be able to register with Pearson VUE and locate a center through the NREMT website.

With the realization of CAT, the NREMT also implemented security measures to ensure the individual taking the exam is the actual paramedic candidate. This security process has been described as extreme. Be prepared for this, so as not to become anxious prior to starting the CAT exam.

Exam administrators will take candidates to a private, secure room. No cell phones are permitted in the room. You will be required to empty your pockets to ensure that they do not contain notes or other prohibited information. Exam administrators also will fingerprint you to confirm identity. In the event that you need to use the restroom, you must call the moderator, who will stop the exam, escort you to the restroom, stand outside the restroom, escort you back to the exam room, and refingerprint you. Do not be alarmed when this occurs, as it is standard procedure for all candidates.

For additional information on what will occur at a Pearson VUE test center, visit the NREMT website at www.nremt.org.

The Paramedic Psychomotor Exam

After a lengthy period of review, revision, and pilot testing in the 1990s, the NREMT presented new practical exam instruments for paramedics in October 2000. The revised advanced-level practical exam is intended to assess the abilities of new paramedics to do their job in an out-of-hospital setting. Skills are assessed via scenarios in which the candidate plays the part of the paramedic.

The NREMT emphasizes that the practical exam is designed not as a teaching instrument but as a testing instrument; the candidate must go into the exam prepared to function as a paramedic, not to learn how to become one. The NREMT's practical tests assess skills in accordance with the 2007 National EMS Scope of Practice Model and the 2009 National Emergency Medical Services Education Standards, as well as current American Heart Association guidelines for Advanced Life Support (ALS) and Basic Cardiac Life Support (BCLS). The NREMT has also developed a Psychomotor Practical Competency Portfolio that continually evaluates the paramedic student through-

out laboratory, clinical, and field internship skills. This portfolio is required prior to sitting for the NREMT cognitive exam and prepares the student for the NREMT Psychomotor Exam.

Paramedic candidates taking the NREMT practical exam are tested on 12 skills:

1. Patient Assessment—Trauma
2. Ventilatory Management—Adult
3. Ventilatory Management—Dual Lumen Airway Device
4. Cardiac Management Skills—Dynamic Cardiology
5. Cardiac Management Skills—Static Cardiology
6. IV and Medication Skills—Intravenous Therapy
7. IV and Medication Skills—Intravenous Bolus Medications
8. Oral Station—Case A
9. Oral Station—Case B
10. Pediatric Skills—Pediatric Ventilatory Management
11. Pediatric Skills—Pediatric Intraosseous Infusion
12. Random Basic Skills, evaluated in one of the following chosen at random: Spinal Immobilization (Seated Patient), Spinal Immobilization (Supine Patient), or Bleeding Control/Shock Management

See Chapter 8 for details about how each of these skills is assessed on the practical exam.

The practical exam is scored pass/fail, with each skill scored separately. If you fail five or fewer skills when taking the whole test, you are entitled to retest up to two times on just those skills you failed. If you fail the second retest (for even one skill), you will be required to take remedial training in all 12 skills. In order to sign up to take the full practical exam (all 12 skills) following remedial training, you will have to provide documentation of completion of remedial training signed by the paramedic training program director or physician medical director of training/ operations for your program. Candidates for paramedic certification who have already passed the NREMT-Intermediate/99 practical exam within the preceding 12 months have a leg up: They can apply the results of the NREMT-Intermediate/99 exam to their first full attempt of the EMT-Paramedic/ Paramedic exam for these four skills:

1. IV and Medication Skills—Intravenous Therapy
2. IV and Medication Skills—Intravenous Bolus Medications
3. Pediatric Skills—Pediatric Intraosseous Infusion
4. Random Basic Skills

If you take this route (applying the four passed EMT-Intermediate/99 skills to your paramedic practical exam), the rules for pass/fail are similar to those just outlined. However, if you fail, and fail both opportunities to retest, you must undergo remedial training in all 12 skills and then take the psychomotor exam on all 12 skills.

No matter the approach, failing six or more skills means the candidate fails the entire psychomotor exam, and that candidate must document remedial training on all 12 skills before retesting. A candidate may take the full psychomotor exam (a test on all 12 skills with two opportunities for retesting on up to five failed skills) a maximum of three times. If a candidate failed the full exam three times, the candidate would have to complete a new state-approved paramedic training program in order to test again.

Using This Book to Prepare

In addition to information about the paramedic practical exam (Chapter 8), this book contains five complete practice tests, each containing 150 items similar to those on the Paramedic cognitive exam. Table 1.1 on page 3 shows the breakdown of content areas in each of the practice tests in this book.

Although some of the questions in these tests provide a scenario followed by a series of questions related to the scenario, this type of question does not appear on the computerized version of the NREMT cognitive exam. We have left them in the practice exams, however, because they require a certain thought process that will help you better prepare for the NREMT exam. In addition, this type of serial scenario questioning often appears on state certification exams.

The first step in using this book to prepare for the EMT-Paramedic/Paramedic cognitive examination is to read Chapter 2, which presents the nine-step LearningExpress Test Preparation System. This chapter provides essential test-taking strategies that you can practice as you take the exams in this book. Next, take one complete practice exam and score your answers using the answer key. Complete explanations of the answers are provided in the Answers section— make use of them! You will not be permitted to use any electronic devices (PDA, calculator, and so forth) while taking the actual exam, so do not use them on the practice tests.

Remember, competency in all content areas is required for successful completion of the CAT exam. If you notice that you are missing a lot of questions in one content area, you should concentrate future studying in that area, in addition to making a comprehensive review of the curriculum in preparation for the actual exam.

As you take each test in this book, pay particular attention to the material at the beginning of each chapter, as we have supplied specific strategies for how to focus with each test. After reading and study-ing this book, you will be well on your way to obtain-ing certification as a paramedic. Good luck as you advance in this rewarding and worthwhile career!

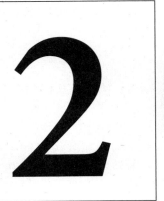

2 ▶ THE LEARNINGEXPRESS TEST PREPARATION SYSTEM

CHAPTER SUMMARY

Taking the Paramedic exam can be tough. It demands a lot of preparation if you want to achieve a top score, and your career in emergency medical services depends on your passing the exam. The LearningExpress Test Preparation System, developed exclusively for LearningExpress by leading test experts, gives you the discipline, attitude, and advantage you need to be a winner.

First, the bad news: Taking the Paramedic exam is no easy feat, and neither is getting ready for it. Your future career as a paramedic depends on your passing the exam, but there are all sorts of pitfalls that can keep you from doing your best. Here are some of the obstacles that can stand in the way of your success:

- Being unfamiliar with the format of the exam
- Being paralyzed by test anxiety
- Leaving your preparation to the last minute
- Not preparing at all!
- Not knowing vital test-taking skills, such as how to pace yourself through the exam, how to use the process of elimination, and when to guess
- Not being in tip-top mental and physical shape
- Arriving late at the test site, working through the test on an empty stomach, or shivering through the exam because the room is cold

What's the common denominator in all these test-taking pitfalls? One word: *control*. Who's in control, you or the exam?

Now the good news: The LearningExpress Test Preparation System puts you in control. In just nine easy-to-follow steps, you will learn everything you need to know to make sure that you are in charge of your preparation and your performance on the exam. Other test takers may let the test get the better of them; other test takers may be unprepared or out of shape, but not you. You will have taken all the steps you need to take to succeed on the Paramedic exam.

Here's how the LearningExpress Test Preparation System works: Nine easy steps lead you through everything you need to know and do to get ready to master your exam. Each of the following steps involves some reading and activities that will help build confidence. It's important that you do the activities along with the reading, or else you won't be getting the full benefit of the system. Each step tells you approximately how much time that step will take you to complete.

Step 1. Get information		(50 minutes)
Step 2. Conquer test anxiety		(20 minutes)
Step 3. Make a plan		(30 minutes)
Step 4. Learn to manage your time		(10 minutes)
Step 5. Learn to use the process of elimination		(20 minutes)
Step 6. Know when to guess		(20 minutes)
Step 7. Reach your peak performance zone		(10 minutes)
Step 8. Get your act together		(10 minutes)
Step 9. Do it!		(10 minutes)
Total		**(3 hours)**

We estimate that working through the entire system will take you approximately three hours, although it's perfectly okay if you work faster or slower than the time estimates assume. If you can take a whole afternoon or evening, you can work through the whole LearningExpress Test Preparation System in one sitting. Otherwise, you can break it up and do just one or two steps a day for the next several days. It's up to you—remember, you're in control.

Step 1: Get Information

Time to complete: 50 minutes
Activities: Read Chapter 1, "About the Paramedic Exam," and Chapter 9, "State Certification Requirements."

Knowledge is power. The first step in the LearningExpress Test Preparation System is finding out everything you can about the Paramedic exam. Once you have your information, the next steps in the LearningExpress Test Preparation System will show you what to do with it.

Part A: Straight Talk about the Paramedic Exam

Why do you have to take this exam, anyway? Simply put, because lives depend on your performance in the field. The Paramedic cognitive exam is just one part of a whole series of evaluations you have to go through to show that you can be trusted with the health and safety of the people you serve. The cognitive exam attempts to measure your knowledge of your trade. The practical skills exam attempts to measure your ability to apply what you know.

It's important for you to realize that your score on the Paramedic cognitive exam does not determine how smart you are or even whether you will make a good paramedic. There are all kinds of things an exam like this can't test: whether you are likely to show up late or call in sick a lot, whether you can keep your cool under the stress of trying to revive a victim of cardiac arrest, whether you can be trusted with confidential information about people's health. Those kinds of things are hard to evaluate, while whether you can click on the right answer is easy to evaluate.

This is not to say that clicking on the right answer is not important! The knowledge tested on the cognitive exam is knowledge you will need to do your job. And your ability to enter the profession you've trained for depends on your passing this exam. And that's why you're here—using the LearningExpress Test Preparation System to achieve control over the exam.

Part B: What's on the Test

If you haven't already done so, stop here and read Chapter 1 of this book, which gives you an overview of Paramedic cognitive exams in general and the National Registry of Emergency Medical Technicians (NREMT) exam in particular.

Many states use the NREMT exam, but others do not. Turn to Chapter 9 for a state-by-state overview of certification requirements. If you haven't already received the full rundown on certification procedures as part of your training program, you can contact the state EMS agency listed in Chapter 9 for details.

Step 2: Conquer Test Anxiety

Time to complete: 20 minutes
Activity: Take the Test Anxiety Quiz.

Having complete information about the exam is the first step in getting control of it. Next, you have to overcome one of the biggest obstacles to test suc-

cess: anxiety. Test anxiety can not only impair your performance on the exam itself, but it can even keep you from preparing! In Step 2, you'll learn stress-management techniques that will help you succeed on your exam. Learn these strategies now and practice them as you work through the exams in this book, so they'll be second nature to you by exam day.

Combating Test Anxiety

The first thing you need to know is that a little test anxiety is a good thing. Everyone gets nervous before a big exam—and if that nervousness motivates you to prepare thoroughly, so much the better. It's said that Sir Laurence Olivier, one of the foremost British actors of last century, was ill before every performance. His stage fright didn't impair his performance; in fact, it probably gave him a little extra edge—just the kind of edge you need to do well, whether on a stage or in an exam room.

On page 13 is the Test Anxiety Quiz. Stop here and answer the questions on that page to find out whether your level of test anxiety is something you should worry about.

Stress Management before the Test

If you feel your level of anxiety getting the best of you in the weeks before the test, here is what you need to do to bring the level down again:

- **Get prepared.** There's nothing like knowing what to expect. Being prepared will put you in control of test anxiety. That's why you are reading this book. Use it faithfully, and remind yourself that you're better prepared than most of the people taking the test.

- **Practice self-confidence.** A positive attitude is a great way to combat test anxiety. This is no time to be humble or shy. Stand in front of the mirror and say to your reflection, "I'm prepared. I'm full of self-confidence. I'm going to ace this test. I know I can do it." Say it into a recording device and play it back once a day. If you hear it often enough, you'll believe it.
- **Fight negative messages.** Every time someone starts telling you how hard the exam is or how it's almost impossible to get a high score, start telling them your self-confidence messages. If you are telling yourself you don't do well on exams or that you just can't do this, don't listen. Turn on your tape recorder and listen to your self-confidence messages.
- **Visualize.** Imagine yourself reporting for duty on your first day as a paramedic. Think of yourself responding to calls, interacting with patients, preserving health, and saving lives. Visualizing success can help make it happen—and it reminds you of why you're doing all this work preparing for the exam.
- **Exercise.** Physical activity helps calm your body down and focus your mind. Besides, being in good physical shape can actually help you do well on the exam. Go for a run, lift weights, go swimming—and do it regularly.

Stress Management on Test Day

There are several ways you can bring down your level of test anxiety on test day. They'll work best if you practice them in the weeks before the test, so you know which ones work best for you:

- **Deep breathing.** Take a deep breath while you count to five. Hold it on the count of one, and then let it out on the count of five. Repeat several times.

- **Move your body.** Try rolling your head in a circle. Rotate your shoulders. Shake your hands from the wrist. Many people find these movements very relaxing.
- **Visualize again.** Think of the place where you are most relaxed: lying on the beach in the sun, walking through the park, or whatever. Now close your eyes and imagine you're actually there. If you practice in advance, you'll find that you only need a few seconds of this exercise to experience a significant increase in your sense of well-being.

When anxiety threatens to overwhelm you right there during the exam, there are still things you can do to manage the stress level:

- **Repeat your self-confidence messages.** You should have them memorized by now. Say them quietly to yourself, and believe them!
- **Visualize one more time.** This time, visualize yourself moving smoothly and quickly through the test, answering every question correctly, and finishing just before time is up. Like most visualization techniques, this one works best if you've practiced it ahead of time.
- **Find an easy question.** Skim over the test until you find an easy question, and answer it. Filling in even one circle gets you into the test-taking groove.
- **Take a mental break.** Everyone loses concentration once in a while during a long test. It's normal, so you shouldn't worry about it. Instead, accept what has happened. Say to yourself, "Hey, I lost it there for a minute. My brain is taking a break." Put down your pencil, close your eyes, and do some deep breathing for a few seconds. Then you're ready to go back to work.

Try these techniques ahead of time, and see if they work for you!

You need to worry about test anxiety only if it is extreme enough to impair your performance. The following questionnaire will provide a diagnosis of your level of test anxiety. In the blank before each statement, write the number that most accurately describes your experience.

0 = Never   1 = Once or twice   2 = Sometimes   3 = Often

_____ I have gotten so nervous before an exam that I simply put down the books and didn't study for it.

_____ I have experienced disabling physical symptoms such as vomiting and severe headaches because I was nervous about an exam.

_____ I have simply not showed up for an exam because I was scared to take it.

_____ I have experienced dizziness and disorientation while taking an exam.

_____ I have had trouble filling in the little circles because my hands were shaking too hard.

_____ I have failed an exam because I was too nervous to complete it.

_____ **Total: Add up the numbers in the blanks above.**

Your Test Anxiety Score

Here are the steps you should take, depending on your score. If you scored:

- **Below 3,** your level of test anxiety is nothing to worry about; it's probably just enough to give you that little extra edge.

- **Between 3 and 6,** your test anxiety may be enough to impair your performance, and you should practice the stress management techniques listed in this chapter to try to bring your test anxiety down to manageable levels.

- **Above 6,** your level of test anxiety is a serious concern. In addition to practicing the stress management techniques listed in this chapter, you may want to seek additional, personal help. Call your local high school or community college and ask for the academic counselor. Tell the counselor that you have a level of test anxiety that sometimes keeps you from being able to take the exam. The counselor may be willing to help you or may suggest someone else you should talk to.

Step 3: Make a Plan

Time to complete: 30 minutes
Activity: Construct a study plan.

Maybe the most important thing you can do to get control of yourself and your exam is to make a study plan. Too many people fail to prepare simply because they fail to plan. Spending hours on the day before the exam poring over sample test questions not only raises your level of test anxiety, but also is no substitute for careful preparation over time.

Don't fall into the cram trap. Take control of your preparation time by mapping out a study schedule. On the following pages are two sample schedules, based on the amount of time you have before you take the Paramedic cognitive exam. If you're the kind of person who needs deadlines and assignments to motivate you for a project, here they are. If you're the kind of person who doesn't like to follow other people's plans, you can use the suggested schedules here to construct your own.

Even more important than making a plan is making a commitment. You can't review everything you learned in your paramedic course in one night. You have to set aside some time every day for study and practice. Try for at least 20 minutes a day. Twenty minutes daily will do you much more good than two hours on Saturday.

Don't put off your studying until the day before the exam. Start now. A few minutes a day, with half an hour or more on weekends, can make a big difference in your score.

Step 4: Learn to Manage Your Time

Time to complete: 10 minutes to read; many hours of practice!
Activities: Practice these strategies as you take the sample tests in this book.

Steps 4, 5, and 6 of the LearningExpress Test Preparation System put you in charge of your exam by showing you test-taking strategies that work. Practice these strategies as you take the sample tests in this book, and then you'll be ready to use them on test day.

First, you'll take control of your time on the exam. Paramedic exams have a two-and-a-half hour time limit, which may give you more than enough time to complete all the questions—or may not. Here are some tips to keep that from happening to you.

- **Follow directions.** If the directions are given orally, listen to them. Ask questions *before* the exam begins if there's anything you don't understand.
- **Read the entire first question.** You should read the whole question first at least twice and formulate the answer in your head before you look at the answer choices. If you look at the answer choices *before* you understand the question, you might choose incorrectly.
- **Look out for qualifiers.** Take note of words like *except*, *always*, *never*, or *most appropriate*. These words limit the potential answers and can help you determine an answer more efficiently.

If you have at least a month before you take the Paramedic exam, you have plenty of time to prepare—as long as you don't waste it! If you have less than a month, turn to Schedule B.

Time	Preparation
Days 1–4	Skim over the written materials from your training program, particularly noting (1) areas you expect to be emphasized on the exam and (2) areas you don't remember well. On Day 4, concentrate on those areas.
Day 5	Take the practice exam in Chapter 3.
Day 6	Score the first practice exam. Use the outline of skills in Table 1.1 on page 3 to determine your strongest and weakest areas. Identify two areas that you will concentrate on before you take the second practice exam.
Days 7–10	Study the two areas you identified as your weak points. Don't worry about the other areas.
Day 11	Take the second practice exam in Chapter 4.
Day 12	Score the second practice exam. Identify one area to concentrate on before you take the third practice exam.
Days 13–18	Study the one area you identified for review. In addition, review both practice exams you've taken so far, with special attention to the answer explanations.
Day 19	Take the third practice exam in Chapter 5.
Day 20	Once again, identify one area to review, based on your score on the third practice exam.
Days 20–21	Study the one area you identified for review.
Days 22–25	Take an overview of all your training materials, consolidating your strengths and improving on your weaknesses.
Day 26	Review all the areas that have given you the most trouble in the three practice exams you've taken so far.
Days 27–28	Take the fourth practice exam in Chapter 6 and score it. Then take the fifth practice exam. Note how much you've improved!
Day 29	Review one or two weak areas.
Day before the exam	Relax. Do something unrelated to the exam and go to bed at a reasonable hour.

SCHEDULE B: THE 10-DAY PLAN

If you have two weeks or less before you take the exam, you may have your work cut out for you. Use this 10-day schedule to help you make the most of your time.

Time	Preparation
Day 1	Take the first practice exam in Chapter 3 and score it using the answer key at the end. Turn to the list of subject areas in Table 1.1 on page 3, and find out which areas need the most work, based on your exam score.
Day 2	Review one area that gave you trouble on the first practice exam.
Day 3	Review another area that gave you trouble on the first practice exam.
Day 4	Take the second practice exam in Chapter 4 and score it.
Day 5	If your second score on the second practice exam doesn't show improvement on the two areas you studied, review them. If you did improve in those areas, choose a new weak area to study today.
Day 6	Take the third practice exam in Chapter 5 and score it.
Day 7	Choose your weakest area from your third practice exam to review. Review any areas that you have not yet reviewed in this schedule.
Day 8	Take the fourth practice exam in Chapter 6 and score it. Review your weakest areas once again.
Day 9	Take the fifth practice exam in Chapter 7 and score it. Brush up on any areas that are still giving you trouble.
Day 10	Use your last study day to brush up on any areas that are still giving you trouble.
Day before the exam	Relax. Do something unrelated to the exam and go to bed at a reasonable hour.

- **Keep moving.** Don't waste time on one question for too long. Remember, though, once you skip a question you cannot come back to it later.
- **Do not make questions more complicated than they are.** You should not bring elements into a question that are not there. This will cause you to overlook the basics, which is probably what the question is testing.
- **Don't rush.** Although you should keep moving, rushing won't help. Try to keep calm and work methodically and quickly.

Step 5: Learn to Use the Process of Elimination

Time to complete: 20 minutes
Activity: Complete worksheet on Using the Process of Elimination.

After time management, your next most important tool for taking control of your exam is using the process of elimination wisely. It's standard test-taking wisdom that you should always read all the answer choices before choosing your answer. This helps you find the right answer by eliminating wrong answer choices. And, sure enough, that standard wisdom applies to your exam, too.

Let's say you're facing a question that goes like this:

13. Which of the following lists of signs and symptoms indicates cardiac compromise?
    a. headache, dizziness, nausea, confusion
    b. dull chest pain, sudden sweating, difficulty breathing
    c. wheezing, labored breathing, chest pain
    d. difficulty breathing, high fever, rapid pulse

You should always use the process of elimination on a question like this, even if the right answer jumps out at you. Sometimes, the answer that jumps out isn't right after all. Let's assume, for the purpose of this exercise, that you're a little rusty on your signs and symptoms of cardiac compromise, so you need to use a little intuition to make up for what you don't remember. Proceed through the answer choices in order.

So you start with choice **a**. This one is pretty easy to eliminate; none of these signs and symptoms is consistent with cardiac compromise.

On to the next. "Dull chest pain" looks good, though if you're not up on your cardiac signs and symptoms, you might wonder if it should be "acute chest pain" instead. "Sudden sweating" and "difficulty breathing"? Check. Make the following mental note: "Good answer, I might use this one."

Choice **c**, is a possibility. Maybe you don't really expect wheezing in cardiac compromise, but you know "chest pain" is right, and let's say you're not sure whether "labored breathing" is a sign of cardiac difficulty. In your head, put a question mark next to **c**, meaning "Well, maybe."

Choice **d** strikes you about the same, with "difficulty breathing" being a good sign of cardiac compromise. But wait a minute. "High fever"? Not really. "Rapid pulse"? Well, maybe. This doesn't really sound like cardiac compromise, and you've already got a better answer picked out in choice **b**. If you're feeling sure of yourself, mentally put an **X** next to this one. If you want to be careful, put a question mark.

In your head, your question looks like this:

13. Which of the following lists of signs and symptoms indicates cardiac compromise?

   X **a.** headache, dizziness, nausea, confusion

   ✓ **b.** dull chest pain, sudden sweating, difficulty breathing

   ? **c.** wheezing, labored breathing, chest pain

   ? **d.** difficulty breathing, high fever, rapid pulse

You've got just one good answer. If you're pressed for time, you should simply select choice **b**. If you've got the time to be extra careful, you could compare your good answer to your question mark answers to make sure that it's better.

It's good to have a system for marking good, bad, and maybe answers. We're recommending this one:

   X = bad

   ✓ = good

   ? = maybe

If you don't like these marks, devise your own system. Just make sure you do it long before test day—while you're working through the practice tests in this book—so you won't have to worry about it during the actual exam.

Even when you think you're absolutely clueless about a question, you can often use the process of elimination to get rid of one answer choice. If so, you're better prepared to make an educated guess, as you'll see in Step 6. More often, the process of elimination allows you to get down to only two possibly right answers. Then you're in a strong position to guess. And sometimes, even though you don't know the right answer, you find it simply by getting rid of the wrong ones, as you did in the previous example.

Try using your powers of elimination on the questions in the Using the Process of Elimination worksheet beginning on the next page. The answer explanations for this worksheet show one way you might use the process to arrive at the right answer.

The process of elimination is your tool for the next step, which is knowing when to guess.

USING THE PROCESS OF ELIMINATION

Use the process of elimination to answer the following questions.

1. Ilsa is as old as Meghan will be in five years. The difference between Ed's age and Meghan's age is twice the difference between Ilsa's age and Meghan's age. Ed is 29. How old is Ilsa?
   a. 4
   b. 10
   c. 19
   d. 24

2. "All drivers of commercial vehicles must carry a valid commercial driver's license whenever operating a commercial vehicle."
   According to this sentence, which of the following people need NOT carry a commercial driver's license?
   a. a truck driver idling his engine while waiting to be directed to a loading dock
   b. a bus operator backing her bus out of the way of another bus in the bus lot
   c. a taxi driver driving his personal car to the grocery store
   d. a limousine driver taking the limousine to her home after dropping off her last passenger of the evening

3. Smoking tobacco has been linked to
   a. increased risk of stroke and heart attack.
   b. all forms of respiratory disease.
   c. increasing mortality rates over the past ten years.
   d. juvenile delinquency.

4. Which of the following words is spelled correctly?
   a. incorrigible
   b. outragous
   c. domestickated
   d. understandible

Answers

Here are the answers, as well as some suggestions as to how you might have used the process of elimination to find them.

1. d. You should have eliminated choice **a** off the bat. Ilsa can't be four years old if Meghan is going to be Ilsa's age in five years. The best way to eliminate other answer choices is to try plugging them in to the information given in the problem. For instance, for choice **b**, if Ilsa is 10, then Meghan must be 5. The difference in their ages is 5. The difference between Ed's age, 29, and Meghan's age, 5, is 24. Is 24 two times 5? No. Then choice **b** is wrong. You could eliminate choice **c** in the same way and be left with choice **d**.

2. c. Note the word *not* in the question, and go through the answers one by one. Is the truck driver in choice **a** "operating a commercial vehicle"? Yes, idling counts as "operating," so he needs to have a commercial driver's license. Likewise, the bus operator in choice **b** is operating a commercial vehicle; the question doesn't say the operator has to be on the street. The limo driver in choice **d** is operating a commercial vehicle, even if it doesn't have a passenger in it. However, the cabbie in choice **c** is not operating a commercial vehicle, but his own private car.

3. a. You could eliminate choice **b** simply because of the presence of the word *all*. Such absolutes hardly ever appear in correct answer choices. Choice **c** looks attractive until you think a little about what you know—aren't fewer people smoking these days, rather than more? So how could smoking be responsible for a higher mortality rate? (If you didn't know that mortality rate means the rate at which people die, you might keep this choice as a possibility, but you would still be able to eliminate two answers and have only two to choose from.) And choice **d** is unlikely, so you could eliminate that one, too. You are left with the correct choice, **a**.

4. a. How you used the process of elimination here depends on which words you recognized as being spelled incorrectly. If you knew that the correct spellings were *outrageous*, *domesticated*, and *understandable*, then you were home free.

Step 6: Know When to Guess

Time to complete: 20 minutes
Activity: Complete the worksheet on Your Guessing Ability.

Armed with the process of elimination, you're ready to take control of one of the big questions in test taking: Should I guess? The first and main answer is *yes*. Some exams have what's called a "guessing penalty," in which a fraction of your wrong answers is subtracted from your right answers—but the Paramedic exam does not work like that. The number of questions you answer correctly yields your competency or incompetency. So you have nothing to lose and everything to gain by guessing.

The more complicated answer to the question, "Should I guess?" depends on you—your personality and your "guessing intuition." There are two things you need to know about yourself before you go into the exam:

- Are you a risk taker?
- Are you a good guesser?

You'll have to decide about your risk-taking quotient on your own. To find out if you're a good guesser, complete the Your Guessing Ability worksheet that begins on page 21. Frankly, even if you're a play-it-safe person with terrible intuition, you're still safe in guessing every time. The best thing would be if you could overcome your anxieties and go ahead and pick an answer. But you may want to have a sense of how good your intuition is before you go into the exam.

Step 7: Reach Your Peak Performance Zone

Time to complete: 10 minutes to read; weeks to complete!
Activity: Complete the Physical Preparation Checklist.

To get ready for a challenge like a big exam, you have to take control of your physical, as well as your mental state. Exercise, proper diet, and rest will ensure that your body works with, rather than against, your mind on test day, as well as during your preparation.

Exercise

If you don't already have a regular exercise program going, the time during which you're preparing for an exam is actually an excellent time to start one. You'll have to be pretty fit to pass your physical ability test anyway. And if you are already keeping fit—or trying to get that way—don't let the pressure of preparing for an exam fool you into quitting now. Exercise helps reduce stress by pumping wonderful good-feeling hormones called endorphins into your system. It also increases the oxygen supply throughout your body and your brain, so you'll be at peak performance on test day.

A half hour of vigorous activity—enough to raise a sweat—every day should be your aim. If you are really pressed for time, every other day is okay. Choose an activity you like and get out there and do it. Jogging with a friend always makes the time go faster, as does listening to music.

But don't overdo it. You don't want to exhaust yourself. Moderation is the key.

YOUR GUESSING ABILITY

The following are ten really hard questions. You are not supposed to know the answers. Rather, this is an assessment of your ability to guess when you don't have a clue. Read each question carefully, just as if you did expect to answer it. If you have any knowledge of the subject, use that knowledge to help you eliminate wrong answer choices.

1. ⓐ ⓑ ⓒ ⓓ
2. ⓐ ⓑ ⓒ ⓓ
3. ⓐ ⓑ ⓒ ⓓ
4. ⓐ ⓑ ⓒ ⓓ
5. ⓐ ⓑ ⓒ ⓓ
6. ⓐ ⓑ ⓒ ⓓ
7. ⓐ ⓑ ⓒ ⓓ
8. ⓐ ⓑ ⓒ ⓓ
9. ⓐ ⓑ ⓒ ⓓ
10. ⓐ ⓑ ⓒ ⓓ

1. September 7 is Independence Day in
   a. India.
   b. Costa Rica.
   c. Brazil.
   d. Australia.

2. Which of the following is the formula for determining the momentum of an object?
   a. $p = mv$
   b. $F = ma$
   c. $P = IV$
   d. $E = mc^2$

3. Because of the expansion of the universe, the stars and other celestial bodies are all moving away from each other. This phenomenon is known as
   a. Newton's first law.
   b. the big bang.
   c. gravitational collapse.
   d. Hubble flow.

4. American author Gertrude Stein was born in
   a. 1713.
   b. 1830.
   c. 1874.
   d. 1901.

5. Which of the following is NOT one of the Five Classics attributed to Confucius?
   a. *I Ching*
   b. *Book of Holiness*
   c. *Spring and Autumn Annals*
   d. *Book of History*

6. The religious and philosophical doctrine that holds that the universe is constantly in a struggle between good and evil is known as
   a. Pelagianism.
   b. Manichaeism.
   c. neo-Hegelianism.
   d. Epicureanism.

7. The third chief justice of the U.S. Supreme Court was
   a. John Blair.
   b. William Cushing.
   c. James Wilson.
   d. John Jay.

8. Which of the following is the poisonous portion of a daffodil?
   a. the bulb
   b. the leaves
   c. the stem
   d. the flowers

9. The winner of the Masters golf tournament in 1953 was
   a. Sam Snead.
   b. Cary Middlecoff.
   c. Arnold Palmer.
   d. Ben Hogan.

10. The state with the highest per capita personal income in 1980 was
    a. Alaska.
    b. Connecticut.
    c. New York.
    d. Texas.

Answers

Check your answers against the following correct answers.

1. c.
2. a.
3. d.
4. c.
5. b.
6. b.
7. b.
8. a.
9. d.
10. a.

How Did You Do?

You may have simply gotten lucky and actually known the answers to one or two questions. In addition, your guessing was probably more successful if you were able to use the process of elimination on any of the questions. Maybe you didn't know who the third chief justice was (question 7), but you knew that John Jay was the first. In that case, you would have eliminated choice **d** and therefore improved your odds of guessing right from one in four to one in three.

According to probability, you should get two and a half answers correct, so getting either two or three right would be average. If you got four or more right, you may be a really terrific guesser. If you got one or none right, you may be a poor guesser.

Keep in mind, though, that this is only a small sample. You should continue to keep track of your guessing ability as you work through the sample questions in this book. Circle the numbers of questions you guess on as you make your guess; or, if you don't have time while you take the practice tests, go back afterward and try to remember which questions you guessed at. Remember, on a test with four answer choices, your chance of guessing correctly is one in four. So keep a separate "guessing" score for each exam. How many questions did you guess on? How many did you get right? If the number you got right is at least one-fourth of the number of questions you guessed on, you are at least an average guesser—maybe better—and you should always go ahead and guess on the real exam. If the number you got right is significantly lower than one-fourth of the number you guessed on, you would be safe in guessing anyway, but maybe you would feel more comfortable if you guessed only selectively, when you can eliminate a wrong answer or at least have a good feeling about one of the answer choices.

Because the Paramedic exams have no guessing penalty, even if you are a play-it-safe person with lousy intuition, you are still safe guessing every time.

Diet

First of all, cut out the junk. Go easy on caffeine and nicotine, and eliminate alcohol and any other drugs from your system at least two weeks before the exam. Promise to treat yourself the night after the exam, if need be.

What your body needs for peak performance is simply a balanced diet. Eat plenty of fruits and vegetables, along with protein and carbohydrates. Foods that are high in lecithin (an amino acid), such as fish and beans, are especially good brain foods.

The night before the exam, you might "carbo-load" the way athletes do before a contest. Eat a big plate of spaghetti, rice and beans, or whatever your favorite carbohydrate is.

Rest

You probably know how much sleep you need every night to be at your best, even if you don't always get it. Make sure you do get that much sleep, though, for at least a week before the exam. Moderation is important here, too. Extra sleep will just make you groggy.

If you are not a morning person and your exam will be given in the morning, you should reset your internal clock so that your body doesn't think you are taking an exam at 3 A.M. You have to start this process well before the exam. Here's how it works: Get up half an hour earlier each morning, and then go to bed half an hour earlier that night. Don't try it the other way around; you will just toss and turn if you go to bed early without having gotten up early. The next morning, get up another half an hour earlier, and so on. How long you will have to do this depends on how late you are used to getting up. Use the Physical Preparation Checklist on page 24 to make sure you're in tip-top form.

Step 8: Get Your Act Together

Time to complete: 10 minutes to read; time to complete will vary.
Activity: Complete Final Preparations worksheet.

You're in control of your mind and body, you're in charge of test anxiety, your preparation, and your test-taking strategies. Now it's time to take charge of external factors, such as the testing site and the materials you need to take the exam.

Find Out Where the Test Is and Make a Trial Run

The testing agency or your EMS instructor will notify you when and where your exam is being held. Do you know how to get to the testing site? Do you know how long it will take to get there? If not, make a trial run, preferably on the same day of the week at the same time of day. Make note, on the Final Preparations worksheet on page 25, of the amount of time it will take you to get to the exam site. Plan on arriving 10–15 minutes early so you can get the lay of the land, use the bathroom, and calm down. Then figure out how early you will have to get up that morning, and make sure you get up that early every day for a week before the exam.

Gather Your Materials

The night before the exam, lay out the clothes you will wear and the materials you have to bring with you to the exam. Plan on dressing in layers; you won't have any control over the temperature of the examination room. Have a sweater or jacket you can take off if it's warm. Use the checklist on the Final Preparations worksheet on page 25 to help you pull together what you'll need.

Don't Skip Breakfast

Even if you don't usually eat breakfast, do so on exam morning. A cup of coffee doesn't count. Don't eat doughnuts or other sweet foods, either. A sugar high will leave you with a sugar low in the middle of the exam. A mix of protein and carbohydrates is best: Cereal with milk and just a little sugar or eggs with toast will do your body a world of good.

PHYSICAL PREPARATION CHECKLIST

For the week before the test, write down what physical exercise you engaged in and for how long, and what you ate for each meal. Remember, you're trying for at least half an hour of exercise every other day (preferably every day) and a balanced diet that's light on junk food.

Exam minus 7 days

Exercise: _____ for _____ minutes
Breakfast: _____
Lunch: _____
Dinner: _____
Snacks: _____

Exam minus 6 days

Exercise: _____ for _____ minutes
Breakfast: _____
Lunch: _____
Dinner: _____
Snacks: _____

Exam minus 5 days

Exercise: _____ for _____ minutes
Breakfast: _____
Lunch: _____
Dinner: _____
Snacks: _____

Exam minus 4 days

Exercise: _____ for _____ minutes
Breakfast: _____
Lunch: _____
Dinner: _____
Snacks: _____

Exam minus 3 days

Exercise: _____ for _____ minutes
Breakfast: _____
Lunch: _____
Dinner: _____
Snacks: _____

Exam minus 2 days

Exercise: _____ for _____ minutes
Breakfast: _____
Lunch: _____
Dinner: _____
Snacks: _____

Exam minus 1 day

Exercise: _____ for _____ minutes
Breakfast: _____
Lunch: _____
Dinner: _____
Snacks: _____

Getting to the Exam Site

Location of exam site: _____

Date: _____

Departure time: _____

Do I know how to get to the exam site?   Yes ___   No ___   (If no, make a trial run.)

Time it will take to get to exam site: _____

Things to Lay Out the Night Before

Clothes I will wear   ___

Sweater/jacket   ___

Watch   ___

Photo ID (*one form for CMA; two forms for RMA*)   ___

Four #2 pencils (*if taking paper-based exam*)   ___

Scheduling permit (*for CMA exam only*)   ___

Other Things to Bring/Remember

_____   _____

_____   _____

_____   _____

_____   _____

Step 9: Do It!

Time to complete: 10 minutes, plus test-taking time
Activity: Ace the Paramedic exam!

Fast forward to exam day. You are ready. You made a study plan and followed through. You practiced your test-taking strategies while working through this book. You are in control of your physical, mental, and emotional state. You know when and where to show up and what to bring with you. In other words, you're better prepared than most of the other people taking the Paramedic exam with you. You are psyched!

Just one more thing. When you're done with the exam, you will have earned a reward. Plan a celebration. Call your friends and plan a party, or have a nice dinner for two—whatever your heart desires. Give yourself something to look forward to.

And then do it. Go into the exam, full of confidence, armed with test-taking strategies you have practiced until they are second nature. You are in control of yourself, your environment, and your performance on exam day. You are ready to succeed. So do it. Go in there and ace the exam! And, then, look forward to your future career as a paramedic!

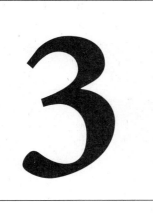

3 ▶ PARAMEDIC PRACTICE EXAM 1

CHAPTER SUMMARY

This is the first of five practice exams in this book based on the Paramedic cognitive exam. Use this test to find out how much you remember from your training program and where your strengths and weaknesses lie.

Take this first exam in as relaxed a manner as you can, without worrying about timing. You can time yourself on the other exams. You should, however, make sure that you have enough time to take the entire exam in one sitting—at least two hours. Find a quiet place where you can work without being interrupted.

You should use the answer sheet on the following page when taking the test. The correct answers, each fully explained, come after the test. When you have read and understood the answer explanations, continue to the end of Chapter 3 for an explanation of how to score your exam.

1.	ⓐ	ⓑ	ⓒ	ⓓ	51.	ⓐ	ⓑ	ⓒ	ⓓ	101.	ⓐ	ⓑ	ⓒ	ⓓ
2.	ⓐ	ⓑ	ⓒ	ⓓ	52.	ⓐ	ⓑ	ⓒ	ⓓ	102.	ⓐ	ⓑ	ⓒ	ⓓ
3.	ⓐ	ⓑ	ⓒ	ⓓ	53.	ⓐ	ⓑ	ⓒ	ⓓ	103.	ⓐ	ⓑ	ⓒ	ⓓ
4.	ⓐ	ⓑ	ⓒ	ⓓ	54.	ⓐ	ⓑ	ⓒ	ⓓ	104.	ⓐ	ⓑ	ⓒ	ⓓ
5.	ⓐ	ⓑ	ⓒ	ⓓ	55.	ⓐ	ⓑ	ⓒ	ⓓ	105.	ⓐ	ⓑ	ⓒ	ⓓ
6.	ⓐ	ⓑ	ⓒ	ⓓ	56.	ⓐ	ⓑ	ⓒ	ⓓ	106.	ⓐ	ⓑ	ⓒ	ⓓ
7.	ⓐ	ⓑ	ⓒ	ⓓ	57.	ⓐ	ⓑ	ⓒ	ⓓ	107.	ⓐ	ⓑ	ⓒ	ⓓ
8.	ⓐ	ⓑ	ⓒ	ⓓ	58.	ⓐ	ⓑ	ⓒ	ⓓ	108.	ⓐ	ⓑ	ⓒ	ⓓ
9.	ⓐ	ⓑ	ⓒ	ⓓ	59.	ⓐ	ⓑ	ⓒ	ⓓ	109.	ⓐ	ⓑ	ⓒ	ⓓ
10.	ⓐ	ⓑ	ⓒ	ⓓ	60.	ⓐ	ⓑ	ⓒ	ⓓ	110.	ⓐ	ⓑ	ⓒ	ⓓ
11.	ⓐ	ⓑ	ⓒ	ⓓ	61.	ⓐ	ⓑ	ⓒ	ⓓ	111.	ⓐ	ⓑ	ⓒ	ⓓ
12.	ⓐ	ⓑ	ⓒ	ⓓ	62.	ⓐ	ⓑ	ⓒ	ⓓ	112.	ⓐ	ⓑ	ⓒ	ⓓ
13.	ⓐ	ⓑ	ⓒ	ⓓ	63.	ⓐ	ⓑ	ⓒ	ⓓ	113.	ⓐ	ⓑ	ⓒ	ⓓ
14.	ⓐ	ⓑ	ⓒ	ⓓ	64.	ⓐ	ⓑ	ⓒ	ⓓ	114.	ⓐ	ⓑ	ⓒ	ⓓ
15.	ⓐ	ⓑ	ⓒ	ⓓ	65.	ⓐ	ⓑ	ⓒ	ⓓ	115.	ⓐ	ⓑ	ⓒ	ⓓ
16.	ⓐ	ⓑ	ⓒ	ⓓ	66.	ⓐ	ⓑ	ⓒ	ⓓ	116.	ⓐ	ⓑ	ⓒ	ⓓ
17.	ⓐ	ⓑ	ⓒ	ⓓ	67.	ⓐ	ⓑ	ⓒ	ⓓ	117.	ⓐ	ⓑ	ⓒ	ⓓ
18.	ⓐ	ⓑ	ⓒ	ⓓ	68.	ⓐ	ⓑ	ⓒ	ⓓ	118.	ⓐ	ⓑ	ⓒ	ⓓ
19.	ⓐ	ⓑ	ⓒ	ⓓ	69.	ⓐ	ⓑ	ⓒ	ⓓ	119.	ⓐ	ⓑ	ⓒ	ⓓ
20.	ⓐ	ⓑ	ⓒ	ⓓ	70.	ⓐ	ⓑ	ⓒ	ⓓ	120.	ⓐ	ⓑ	ⓒ	ⓓ
21.	ⓐ	ⓑ	ⓒ	ⓓ	71.	ⓐ	ⓑ	ⓒ	ⓓ	121.	ⓐ	ⓑ	ⓒ	ⓓ
22.	ⓐ	ⓑ	ⓒ	ⓓ	72.	ⓐ	ⓑ	ⓒ	ⓓ	122.	ⓐ	ⓑ	ⓒ	ⓓ
23.	ⓐ	ⓑ	ⓒ	ⓓ	73.	ⓐ	ⓑ	ⓒ	ⓓ	123.	ⓐ	ⓑ	ⓒ	ⓓ
24.	ⓐ	ⓑ	ⓒ	ⓓ	74.	ⓐ	ⓑ	ⓒ	ⓓ	124.	ⓐ	ⓑ	ⓒ	ⓓ
25.	ⓐ	ⓑ	ⓒ	ⓓ	75.	ⓐ	ⓑ	ⓒ	ⓓ	125.	ⓐ	ⓑ	ⓒ	ⓓ
26.	ⓐ	ⓑ	ⓒ	ⓓ	76.	ⓐ	ⓑ	ⓒ	ⓓ	126.	ⓐ	ⓑ	ⓒ	ⓓ
27.	ⓐ	ⓑ	ⓒ	ⓓ	77.	ⓐ	ⓑ	ⓒ	ⓓ	127.	ⓐ	ⓑ	ⓒ	ⓓ
28.	ⓐ	ⓑ	ⓒ	ⓓ	78.	ⓐ	ⓑ	ⓒ	ⓓ	128.	ⓐ	ⓑ	ⓒ	ⓓ
29.	ⓐ	ⓑ	ⓒ	ⓓ	79.	ⓐ	ⓑ	ⓒ	ⓓ	129.	ⓐ	ⓑ	ⓒ	ⓓ
30.	ⓐ	ⓑ	ⓒ	ⓓ	80.	ⓐ	ⓑ	ⓒ	ⓓ	130.	ⓐ	ⓑ	ⓒ	ⓓ
31.	ⓐ	ⓑ	ⓒ	ⓓ	81.	ⓐ	ⓑ	ⓒ	ⓓ	131.	ⓐ	ⓑ	ⓒ	ⓓ
32.	ⓐ	ⓑ	ⓒ	ⓓ	82.	ⓐ	ⓑ	ⓒ	ⓓ	132.	ⓐ	ⓑ	ⓒ	ⓓ
33.	ⓐ	ⓑ	ⓒ	ⓓ	83.	ⓐ	ⓑ	ⓒ	ⓓ	133.	ⓐ	ⓑ	ⓒ	ⓓ
34.	ⓐ	ⓑ	ⓒ	ⓓ	84.	ⓐ	ⓑ	ⓒ	ⓓ	134.	ⓐ	ⓑ	ⓒ	ⓓ
35.	ⓐ	ⓑ	ⓒ	ⓓ	85.	ⓐ	ⓑ	ⓒ	ⓓ	135.	ⓐ	ⓑ	ⓒ	ⓓ
36.	ⓐ	ⓑ	ⓒ	ⓓ	86.	ⓐ	ⓑ	ⓒ	ⓓ	136.	ⓐ	ⓑ	ⓒ	ⓓ
37.	ⓐ	ⓑ	ⓒ	ⓓ	87.	ⓐ	ⓑ	ⓒ	ⓓ	137.	ⓐ	ⓑ	ⓒ	ⓓ
38.	ⓐ	ⓑ	ⓒ	ⓓ	88.	ⓐ	ⓑ	ⓒ	ⓓ	138.	ⓐ	ⓑ	ⓒ	ⓓ
39.	ⓐ	ⓑ	ⓒ	ⓓ	89.	ⓐ	ⓑ	ⓒ	ⓓ	139.	ⓐ	ⓑ	ⓒ	ⓓ
40.	ⓐ	ⓑ	ⓒ	ⓓ	90.	ⓐ	ⓑ	ⓒ	ⓓ	140.	ⓐ	ⓑ	ⓒ	ⓓ
41.	ⓐ	ⓑ	ⓒ	ⓓ	91.	ⓐ	ⓑ	ⓒ	ⓓ	141.	ⓐ	ⓑ	ⓒ	ⓓ
42.	ⓐ	ⓑ	ⓒ	ⓓ	92.	ⓐ	ⓑ	ⓒ	ⓓ	142.	ⓐ	ⓑ	ⓒ	ⓓ
43.	ⓐ	ⓑ	ⓒ	ⓓ	93.	ⓐ	ⓑ	ⓒ	ⓓ	143.	ⓐ	ⓑ	ⓒ	ⓓ
44.	ⓐ	ⓑ	ⓒ	ⓓ	94.	ⓐ	ⓑ	ⓒ	ⓓ	144.	ⓐ	ⓑ	ⓒ	ⓓ
45.	ⓐ	ⓑ	ⓒ	ⓓ	95.	ⓐ	ⓑ	ⓒ	ⓓ	145.	ⓐ	ⓑ	ⓒ	ⓓ
46.	ⓐ	ⓑ	ⓒ	ⓓ	96.	ⓐ	ⓑ	ⓒ	ⓓ	146.	ⓐ	ⓑ	ⓒ	ⓓ
47.	ⓐ	ⓑ	ⓒ	ⓓ	97.	ⓐ	ⓑ	ⓒ	ⓓ	147.	ⓐ	ⓑ	ⓒ	ⓓ
48.	ⓐ	ⓑ	ⓒ	ⓓ	98.	ⓐ	ⓑ	ⓒ	ⓓ	148.	ⓐ	ⓑ	ⓒ	ⓓ
49.	ⓐ	ⓑ	ⓒ	ⓓ	99.	ⓐ	ⓑ	ⓒ	ⓓ	149.	ⓐ	ⓑ	ⓒ	ⓓ
50.	ⓐ	ⓑ	ⓒ	ⓓ	100.	ⓐ	ⓑ	ⓒ	ⓓ	150.	ⓐ	ⓑ	ⓒ	ⓓ

Paramedic Exam 1

1. During the initial phase of an acute stress reaction, which of the following physiological responses will occur?
   a. normal vital signs that remain unchanged
   b. increased vital signs that quickly return to normal
   c. increased pulse rate and pupillary dilation
   d. lowered pulse rate and pupillary constriction

2. You use an end-tidal carbon dioxide detector as a tool to determine if endotracheal intubation has been correctly obtained. The absence of carbon dioxide in exhaled air after six ventilations could indicate that the endotracheal tube has been
   a. correctly placed.
   b. placed in the esophagus.
   c. placed in the right mainstem bronchus.
   d. placed in the left mainstem bronchus.

3. The focused history and physical examination of a patient begins after you have
   a. controlled immediate threats to the patient's life.
   b. transported the patient to the hospital.
   c. secured the scene and gained access to the patient.
   d. contacted medical control for direction.

Answer questions 4 and 5 based on the following information.

You arrive on the scene and find an elderly male complaining of severe abdominal and back pain. Upon further questioning, he states that the pain is "all over the left side." On palpation, you feel a pulsating mass in the abdomen.

4. From which of the following is this patient most likely suffering?
   a. pulsating diaphragm lesions
   b. acute arterial occlusion
   c. acute pulmonary embolism
   d. abdominal aortic aneurysm

5. This patient's vital signs have been worsening steadily throughout the time he has been under your care. Which of the following should be included for treatment of this patient?
   a. cardiac monitoring
   b. two liters of crystalloid solution
   c. dopamine administration
   d. PASG/MAST application

6. Which of the following regulates hypoxic drive?
   a. low PaO_2
   b. high PaO_2
   c. high oxygen saturation percentage
   d. low oxygen saturation percentage

7. The posterior tibial pulse can be palpated near which of the following?
   a. arch of the foot
   b. medial ankle bone
   c. posterior knee
   d. top of the foot

8. Which is defined by progressively deeper, faster breathing alternating gradually with shallow, slower breathing?
   a. agonal respiration
   b. Cheyne-Stokes respiration
   c. Kussmaul's respiration
   d. Biot's respiration

9. Which patient should be transported immediately with minimal on-scene care and any attempts at stabilization performed en route to the hospital?
   a. female, 45 years old, P 132 BPM, systolic BP 78 mmHg
   b. male, 60 years old, P 115 BPM, RR 12 breaths per minute
   c. female, 28 years old, systolic BP 96 mmHg, RR 18 breaths per minute
   d. male, 54 years old, P 98 BPM, diastolic BP 80 mmHg

10. Which consists of the collective change in vital signs associated with the late stages of increasing intracranial pressure?
   a. increasing pulse rate, shallow respirations, and increasing blood pressure
   b. slowing pulse rate, deep or erratic respirations, and increasing blood pressure
   c. rapid and shallow pulse, deep respirations, and decreasing blood pressure
   d. quickening pulse rate, shallow respirations, and decreasing blood pressure

11. With which should you treat a patient who has an open abdominal wound with a protruding loop of bowel?
   a. a trauma dressing secured with triangular bandages
   b. an occlusive dressing secured on only three sides
   c. a wet sterile dressing and an occlusive dressing
   d. a clean gauze dressing secured with sterile tape

12. Which of the following patients is most critical in terms of age and mechanism of injury?
   a. an 86-year-old female with a fractured clavicle
   b. a 28-year-old male with a fractured femur
   c. a 43-year-old female with a fractured rib
   d. a 56-year-old male with a pelvic fracture

13. An unconscious patient who has one dilated pupil that is reactive to light is showing early signs of which of the following?
   a. transient ischemic attacks
   b. cerebral artery aneurysm
   c. status epilepticus
   d. increased intracranial pressure

14. Using your sense of touch during a physical examination is called which of the following?
   a. palpation
   b. percussion
   c. palpitation
   d. auscultation

15. A harsh upper-airway sound that can be heard when the patient inhales is called which of the following?
   a. stridor
   b. restriction
   c. dysphonia
   d. dyspnea

16. You suspect that a patient has a complete airway obstruction when he
   a. is wheezing.
   b. cannot cough.
   c. can only whisper.
   d. can exhale only with significant effort.

17. No breath sounds in one lung field may indicate which of the following conditions?
  a. pneumothorax
  b. partial airway obstruction
  c. flail chest
  d. pulmonary embolism

18. Why is ventilating a pediatric patient with a bag-valve mask more difficult than ventilating an adult?
  a. The infant is more combative.
  b. The infant needs a lower concentration of oxygen.
  c. It is more difficult to create a good mask seal in an infant.
  d. The glottic opening is smaller in an infant.

19. The pharyngeal-tracheal lumen (PTL) airway should be removed if the patient does which of the following?
  a. vomits
  b. becomes tachycardic
  c. regains consciousness
  d. has poor compliance

20. A patient with an acute abdomen who shows no signs of hemorrhage and has stable vital signs should be in which of the following positions?
  a. whatever position is most comfortable for the patient
  b. a fetal position with both legs bent
  c. in shock position with both lower legs elevated
  d. sitting upright in a high Fowler's position

21. Which of the following is essential to a focused examination of the abdomen of a patient who is complaining of abdominal pain?
  a. percussion on the entire abdomen
  b. auscultation of the area of discomfort
  c. gentle palpation of the entire abdomen
  d. repeated tests for rebound tenderness

22. Drug dosages are lower in elderly patients than in young adults primarily because elderly patients
  a. weigh less on average than younger patients
  b. have a slower rate of elimination of drugs
  c. forget they took their medication and overdose
  d. do not respond to drugs as well as the young

23. Which set of vital signs is consistent with left heart failure?
  a. BP 100/60 mmHg, P 48 BPM and regular, RR 8 breaths per minute and shallow
  b. BP 130/80 mmHg, P 68 BPM and irregular, RR 14 breaths per minute and normal
  c. BP 160/100 mmHg, P 108 BPM and irregular, RR 26 breaths per minute and labored
  d. BP 170/110 mmHg, P 76 BPM and irregular, RR 22 breaths per minute and shallow

24. Which of the following conditions would NOT result in an increase in a patient's $PaCO_2$?
  a. airway obstruction
  b. hypoventilation
  c. hyperventilation
  d. physical exertion

25. Which of the following is defined as the volume of air normally inhaled or exhaled during each respiration?
  a. tidal volume
  b. total lung capacity
  c. minute volume
  d. inspiratory reserve

Answer questions 26–29 based on the following information.

You are called to the home of an elderly female who is having difficulty breathing. She has a history of chronic congestive heart failure (CHF).

26. Which vital sign pattern does this patient most likely exhibit?
   a. shallow-rapid respirations; decreased pulse rate; cool, clammy skin
   b. deep-labored respirations; decreased pulse rate; hot, dry skin
   c. shallow-rapid respirations; increased pulse rate; cool, clammy skin
   d. increased respiratory rate; decreased pulse rate; flushed, dry skin

27. Which of the following are common medications associated with patients with chronic CHF?
   a. thiamine, nitroglycerine, and albuterol
   b. cortisone, digoxin, and theophylline
   c. furosemide, calcium, and nitroglycerine
   d. diuretics, potassium, and digoxin

28. You auscultate the patient's chest. What lung sounds would you expect to hear from this patient?
   a. basilar wheezes in all lung fields bilaterally
   b. crackles and/or rhonchi mainly in the lower lobes
   c. clear but diminished sounds in the upper lobes
   d. rubs with chest wall expansion in the bases

29. Which of the following best describes the pathophysiology of CHF?
   a. cardiac muscle failure resulting in pulmonary edema
   b. aortic valve failure resulting in pulmonary edema
   c. pneumonia resulting in pulmonary edema
   d. superior vena cava failure resulting in pulmonary edema

30. Overinflating the pilot balloon in an endotracheal tube can cause which of the following?
   a. displacement of the tube
   b. return of the gag reflex
   c. ischemia of the tracheal wall
   d. damage to teeth and gums

31. Which of the following should you perform to ensure proper placement of the endotracheal tube?
   a. Confirm placement of the tube by a minimum of two different methods.
   b. Suction the end of the tube and observe for vomitus or blood.
   c. Check breath sounds in the chest before and after placement.
   d. Visualize the open glottis and remove stylet before tube placement.

32. What does the *T* in DCAP-BTLS stand for?
   a. tenderness
   b. time
   c. tourniquet
   d. trauma

33. Distended neck veins, diminishing unilateral breath sounds, and progressively worsening compliance are indications of which of the following?
   a. esophageal intubation
   b. endobronchial intubation
   c. tension pneumothorax
   d. hemopneumothorax

34. When suctioning a patient, you should always perform which of the following?
 a. Begin suctioning after the catheter is placed in the airway.
 b. Limit suctioning attempts to no more than 45 seconds each.
 c. Hyperventilate the patient after every three suction attempts.
 d. Insert the catheter while the suctioning apparatus is turned on.

35. Your patient exhibits cold, clammy skin; air hunger; distended neck veins; tracheal displacement; and absent breath sounds on one side. You should suspect which of the following?
 a. tension pneumothorax
 b. flail chest
 c. massive hemothorax
 d. pericardial tamponade

36. Which are the signs of circulatory overload in a patient who is receiving IV fluids?
 a. dyspnea, crackles, and rhonchi
 b. agitation and clammy skin
 c. falling blood pressure
 d. trauma score lower than 10

37. What is your first action for an adult patient who is conscious but has a complete airway obstruction?
 a. Deliver rapid abdominal thrusts until cleared or unconsciousness results.
 b. Use the jaw-thrust/chin-lift technique to confirm the obstruction.
 c. Pinch the patient's nostrils and attempt to give two ventilations.
 d. Ask the patient to lie down on the ground and attempt finger sweeps.

38. What is the treatment for someone who is suffering an exacerbation of either emphysema or chronic bronchitis and is not displaying overt signs of hypoxia?
 a. Transport this patient to the hospital rapidly, as there is little care that can be rendered for this condition in the prehospital setting.
 b. Administer high-flow oxygen, establish an IV, place the patient on an ECG monitor, and administer bronchodilators.
 c. Establish an airway, position the patient seated or semiseated, administer low-flow oxygen, establish an IV, and transport.
 d. Establish an airway, administer oxygen at the highest possible concentration, establish an IV, and rapidly transport.

39. What is the most commonly used drug in the prehospital setting for patients with asthma?
 a. IV or intramuscular (IM) corticosteroid
 b. nebulized or subcutaneous (SC) epinephrine
 c. inhaled or nebulized albuterol
 d. IM or IV terbutaline

40. Which one of the following methods is recommended when measuring respiratory rate?
 a. Use a Wright Peak Flow Meter to determine peak expiratory flow rate.
 b. Tell the patient to remain quiet while you count the patient's respirations.
 c. Carry on a conversation with the patient to distract him or her while you count.
 d. Count respirations while pretending to take a radial pulse.

41. You respond to a college fraternity, where you encounter a 19-year-old male with a partially obstructed airway. According to witnesses, he was eating pizza and drinking beer when he began to cough and grab his throat. The patient is only able to speak in a hoarse whisper and he has been coughing repeatedly for about 20 minutes. What is the best treatment for this patient?
    a. Perform abdominal thrusts without back blows.
    b. Administer back blows and chest thrusts.
    c. Remove the obstruction with forceps.
    d. Continuously monitor the patient as he is moving air.

42. To perform a needle cricothyrotomy, you should place the patient in which of the following positions?
    a. supine with head and neck in a slightly flexed position
    b. in the lateral recumbent position with head and neck hyperextended
    c. in the lateral recumbent position with head and neck in a neutral position
    d. supine with head and neck hyperextended

43. Which of the following conditions best suggests respiratory failure?
    a. change in mental status
    b. loud, audible stridor
    c. diaphoresis
    d. tachycardia (> 130)

44. Which of the following can complicate ventilation in a pediatric patient?
    a. hyperextension of the neck
    b. use of an oropharyngeal airway in unconscious patients
    c. a bag-valve mask without a pop-off valve
    d. ventilatory pressure that is higher than is used for adults

45. Which breathing pattern is characterized by periods of apnea followed by periods in which respirations first increase and then decrease in both depth and frequency?
    a. central neurogenic hyperventilation
    b. apneustic respirations
    c. Cheyne-Stokes respiration
    d. diaphragmatic respirations

46. What condition is the pathophysiological result of prolonged immersion in seawater?
    a. ventricular fibrillation
    b. pulmonary edema
    c. pulmonary embolism
    d. metabolic alkalosis

Answer questions 47–51 based on the following information.

You respond along with fire units to the scene of a structure fire. Firefighters have rescued a 25-year-old female who is unconscious and unresponsive to verbal or painful stimuli. The victim was located in a smoke-filled bedroom on the floor above the actual fire. Vital signs are blood pressure 146/80 mmHg; pulse 128 BPM, strong and regular; and respiratory rate 40 breaths per minute. The ECG monitor shows sinus tachycardia. Auscultation reveals generally clear lung sounds and mild expiratory wheezing. You note no burn injuries to the skin or clothing.

47. What would account for the patient's level of consciousness?
   a. She has a drug overdose resulting in unconsciousness.
   b. She has heat stroke from the hot environment.
   c. She is suffering from carbon monoxide poisoning.
   d. She is suffering from carbon dioxide poisoning.

48. Which of the following is the reason why pulse oximetry readings should be scrutinized?
   a. Elevated carbon monoxide levels can cause an inaccurately high reading of the percentage of oxygen saturation.
   b. Elevated carbon monoxide levels can cause an inaccurately low reading of the percentage of oxygen saturation.
   c. Elevated carbon dioxide levels can cause an inaccurately high reading of the percentage of oxygen saturation.
   d. Elevated carbon dioxide levels can cause an inaccurately low reading of the percentage of oxygen saturation.

49. Treatment for carbon monoxide poisoning should include which of the following?
   a. nasal cannula (low-flow) oxygen
   b. IV drip of sodium bicarbonate
   c. transport to a hyperbaric facility
   d. transport in position of comfort

50. Signs of CO exposure include all EXCEPT which one of the following?
   a. cyanotic skin
   b. cherry-red skin
   c. chest pain
   d. hyperactivity

51. Which of the following is a common source of CO?
   a. engine exhaust
   b. cellular respiration
   c. cellular metabolism
   d. well-ventilated space heaters

52. You have arrived on scene to find a 75-year-old female in respiratory distress. Your assessment reveals: BP 138/90 mmHg, P 136 BPM, and RR 34 breaths per minute. Upon auscultation, you note diffuse bilateral wheezes in the apices and diminished breath sounds in the bases. Pulse oximetry is 82% on room air, and the patient appears fatigued. Which of the following treatment guidelines should you follow for this patient?
   1. Establish an IV at a keep veins open (KVO) rate.
   2. Give two 20 mL/kg boluses before establishing an IV at a KVO rate.
   3. If possible, ventilate via BVM at a rate of 24/min. to maximize oxygenation.
   4. Attempt orotracheal or nasotracheal intubation.
   5. Provide oxygen via a nonrebreather mask at 10 lpm.
   a. 1, 3, and 5
   b. 2, 3, and 4
   c. 1, 3, and 4
   d. 1, 3, 4, and 5

53. What is the primary drug for the management of acute anaphylaxis?
   a. diphenhydramine hcl
   b. methylprednisolone
   c. terbutaline
   d. epinephrine

54. You have just started an IV, but the fluid is not flowing properly. What is the first thing you should do to troubleshoot this situation?
  a. Remove the cannula and try another site.
  b. Make sure the constricting band has been removed.
  c. Ensure that the right-size drip set is attached.
  d. Lower the IV bag below the level of the patient's arm.

55. Which of the following patients would benefit most from the application of the PASG/MAST?
  a. 10-year-old male, suspected spinal fracture, no blood loss
  b. 72-year-old female, suspected cardiogenic shock, no blood loss
  c. 40-year-old male, suspected lower extremity fracture, low blood pressure
  d. 67-year-old female, suspected ankle sprain, high blood pressure

56. Care for the patient with cardiac contusion is similar to care for the patient with which of the following conditions?
  a. closed abdominal trauma
  b. pericardial tamponade
  c. tension pneumothorax
  d. myocardial infarction

57. The most common cause of upper-airway obstruction is which of the following?
  a. anaphylaxis
  b. croup
  c. epiglottitis
  d. relaxation of the tongue

58. Fractures and dislocations to the femurs, knees, and hips are common injuries found in frontal automobile collisions with which of the following?
  a. down-and-under pathway
  b. down-and-back pathway
  c. up-and-over pathway
  d. up-and-back pathway

59. What electrical activity occurs within the actual drawing of the QRS complex on an ECG tracing?
  a. only ventricular repolarization
  b. ventricular depolarization and atrial repolarization
  c. ventricular repolarization and atrial depolarization
  d. impulse travel through the atrioventricular junction

60. What does the treatment for a patient whose ECG shows premature atrial contractions include?
  a. observation only as long as the patient remains asymptomatic
  b. vagal maneuvers and 6 mg adenosine rapid IV push over 1–3 seconds
  c. 1–1.5 mg/kg lidocaine via slow IV push, and consider sedation
  d. immediate synchronized cardioversion with 50–100 joules

61. Where does traumatic aortic rupture usually occur as a result of transection of the aorta?
  a. pulmonary artery
  b. ligamentum teres
  c. ligamentum nuchae
  d. ligamentum arteriosum

62. What is the clinical significance of a first-degree AV block?
   a. It signals the onset of rapid cardiovascular decompensation.
   b. It indicates that the heart rate may drop if action is not taken.
   c. It can lead to syncope and angina if not corrected quickly.
   d. It may foreshadow development of a more advanced dysrhythmia.

63. In which situation would you consider having the patient perform a Valsalva maneuver to slow the heart rate?
   a. male, age 34, paroxysmal junctional tachycardia (PJT)
   b. male, age 68, idioventricular escape rhythm
   c. female, age 74, premature ventricular contractions
   d. female, age 39, ventricular tachycardia

64. Which rhythm is likely to foreshadow the development of other, more serious dysrhythmias?
   a. atrial fibrillation
   b. isolated premature atrial contractions
   c. accelerated junctional rhythm
   d. sinus dysrhythmia

65. How should you position the patient to check for jugular vein distention?
   a. lying flat on the patient's back
   b. sitting upright near 90°
   c. standing up in anatomical position
   d. elevated at a 45° angle

66. What does a carotid artery bruit indicate?
   a. good peripheral perfusion
   b. obstruction of blood flow
   c. jugular vein distention
   d. congestive heart failure

67. Hyperextension of the neck, followed by hyperflexion, is common in which of the following?
   a. rear-end impacts
   b. rotational impacts
   c. frontal impacts
   d. lateral impacts

68. The pain of stable angina is brought on by which of the following?
   a. exercise or stress
   b. imminent AMI
   c. difficulty breathing
   d. overuse of nitroglycerin

69. A patient's signs and symptoms include orthopnea, spasmodic coughing, agitation, cyanosis, crackles, jugular vein distention, elevated blood pressure, pulse, and respirations. What condition should you suspect?
   a. left heart failure
   b. right heart failure
   c. myocardial infarction
   d. cardiogenic shock

70. Your patient is exhibiting the signs and symptoms of right-sided heart failure. There is no evidence of left-sided failure. In addition to ECG monitoring and high-flow oxygen, what additional treatments should the patient receive?
   a. IV with minidrip set, dopamine, norepinephrine, and rapid transport
   b. IV with macrodrip set, morphine sulfate, furosemide, and rapid transport
   c. IV with minidrip set, close monitoring of vital signs, and normal transport
   d. IV with macrodrip set, shock position, PASG, and normal transport

71. Which of the following drugs is an antidys-rhythmic agent?
   a. furosemide
   b. lidocaine
   c. nitroglycerin
   d. isoproterenol

72. In performing emergency synchronized cardio-version, you would synchronize the electrical shock with which of the following wave forms?
   a. P wave
   b. R wave
   c. P-R interval
   d. QRS complex

73. Treatment for a patient who is experiencing stable angina consists of
   a. oxygen and defibrillation if the QRS complex is wide.
   b. rest, oxygen, and nitroglycerin administration.
   c. reassurance, oxygen, ECG monitoring, and morphine sulfate.
   d. seating patient upright and starting IV, ECG, and furosemide.

74. The wheezing associated with left-sided heart failure results from which of the following?
   a. fluid in the lungs
   b. chronic bronchitis
   c. chest muscle tightness
   d. chest wall expansion

75. A patient is found in a back bedroom lying supine on the bed with a hunting knife embed-ded in her anterior chest, midline below the right breast. The patient is in obvious respira-tory distress. She is cold, clammy, and diapho-retic with flat neck veins. You hear diminished breath sounds on the right side. This patient most likely is suffering from which of the following?
   a. pneumothorax
   b. pericardial tamponade
   c. tension pneumothorax
   d. hemothorax

76. Which of the following is the most appropriate treatment for an adult patient who has a head injury and is seizing?
   a. 5.0 mg of diazepam IM
   b. 5.0 mg of diazepam IVP
   c. nasal intubation with a 6.5 endotracheal tube
   d. direct laryngoscopy and intubation with a 7.5 endotracheal tube

Answer questions 77–80 based on the following information.

You respond to a 22-year-old male who is com-plaining of a rapid onset of chest pain. The patient states that the pain is tearing and sharp and that it started when he surfaced from a scuba dive from 60 feet down. The patient's diving partner states that the patient surfaced too rapidly.

77. What is this patient most likely suffering from?
   a. acute pulmonary edema
   b. nitrogen narcosis
   c. decompression sickness
   d. pulmonary embolism

78. Treatment for this patient consists of
a. IV, high-flow oxygen, and rapid transport to the nearest emergency department
b. IV, high-flow oxygen, and rapid transport to a recompression chamber
c. IV, orotracheal intubation, and transport to the nearest emergency department
d. IV, orotracheal intubation, and transport to a recompression chamber

79. Due to his rapid ascent, this patient may also be suffering from which other diving-related emergency?
a. nitrogen narcosis
b. acute pulmonary edema
c. decompression sickness
d. pneumonia

80. What is an additional possible problem associated with this injury?
a. an increased level of carbon dioxide in the interstitial spaces
b. nitrogen bubbles entering tissue spaces and smaller blood vessels
c. an increase in oxygen levels in the tracheal-bronchial tree
d. excess accumulation of lactic acid collecting in the alveolar space

81. For which of the following conditions would you be likely to receive an order to administer intravenous thiamine?
a. status epilepticus
b. metabolic shock
c. hyperventilation
d. profound intoxication

82. During delivery, you notice that the amniotic fluid is discolored and has a foul odor. What should you do first?
a. Suction the upper airway using a meconium aspirator.
b. Intubate the child and give positive pressure ventilations.
c. Place the child in a dry and warm position, suction, and stimulate the child to breathe.
d. Provide five back blows and then five chest thrusts.

83. A greenstick fracture is one that is which of the following?
a. open
b. impacted
c. partial
d. comminuted

84. What should you do to care for a patient with a suspected pelvic fracture?
a. Apply a pelvic wrap, titrate two IVs to effect, and monitor for signs of shock.
b. Immobilize the patient to a long spine board, start two IVs, and transport immediately.
c. Gently align lower limbs, apply soft splint with a blanket and cravat, and administer analgesics.
d. Do not immobilize, monitor distal pulse and sensation, and transport immediately.

85. Your patient has a powder chemical burn to her face and eyes. How should you treat this condition?
a. Cover the eyes and face with a dry sterile dressing.
b. Apply a paste made of baking soda and alcohol to the eyes.
c. Apply a neutralizing agent to counteract any chemical reaction.
d. Brush the chemical away and then flush the area with copious amounts of clean cool water.

86. The first step in managing a burn patient is to perform which of the following?
   a. Estimate the percentage and degree of burns.
   b. Assess airway and breathing status.
   c. Prevent contamination by applying sterile burn dressings.
   d. Stop the burning process.

87. A burn wound that blisters is an example of which of the following?
   a. first-degree burn
   b. second-degree burn
   c. third-degree burn
   d. chemical burn

88. An adult who has burns over both sides of one arm and both sides of one leg would be estimated to have burns over what percentage of body surface area?
   a. 9%
   b. 18%
   c. 27%
   d. 36%

89. Your patient is a comatose 56-year-old male. His breath smells fruity and sweet and his respirations are very deep and rapid. After the initial assessment, you should provide which of the following treatments?
   a. Draw blood, start an IV of 0.9% NaCl, and give a 500 mL fluid bolus.
   b. Draw blood, start an IV of normal saline, and administer IM glucagon.
   c. Administer oxygen, start an IV of D5W, and transport immediately.
   d. Administer oxygen, monitor vital signs, and give 25 gm IV dextrose 50%.

90. Signs of hypoglycemia include which of the following?
   a. nausea and vomiting; tachycardia; abdominal pain; deep, rapid respirations
   b. weak, rapid pulse; cold, clammy skin; headache; irritability; coma
   c. shallow, rapid breathing; low blood pressure; warm, dry skin; irritability
   d. decreased blood pressure, pulse, and respirations; loss of consciousness

91. Naloxone is given to patients who are suspected of having which of the following conditions?
   a. narcotic overdose
   b. Wernicke's syndrome
   c. Korsakoff psychosis
   d. increased intracranial pressure

92. Patients who are found in a hazardous-materials incident should be initially treated in which containment zone?
   a. hot
   b. warm
   c. cold
   d. moderate

93. After administration of epinephrine, what may be given to help epinephrine stop an allergic reaction?
   a. oxygen
   b. diphenhydramine
   c. albuterol
   d. terbutaline

94. What is the reason for giving inhaled beta agonists to patients with severe allergic reactions?
   a. to increase heart rate and contractile force
   b. to block histamine receptors so edema is lessened
   c. to help suppress the inflammatory response
   d. to reverse bronchospasm and relax airways

95. A patient is covered with alpha-radioactive material after an accidental spill. An adequate level of shielding would be which of the following?
a. a lead apron
b. a concrete wall
c. a cloth uniform
d. aluminum foil

96. Your patient is a farmer who has employed a crop duster to spray his fields. The fields were sprayed earlier today and now the farmer has teary eyes, nausea and vomiting, diarrhea, and excessive salivation. With what was he most likely poisoned?
a. organophosphates
b. nitrogen-based fertilizer
c. cyanide
d. carbon monoxide

97. Which patient presents the signs and symptoms of moderate hypothermia?
a. male, age 34, core temperature 85.8°F
b. female, age 28, core temperature 88.8°F
c. female, age 47, core temperature 95.8°F
d. male, age 39, core temperature 96.4°F

98. What is the correct field treatment for a frost-bitten body part?
a. Transport the patient to the hospital.
b. Rub the affected part with crushed ice or snow until warmed.
c. Warm the affected part in water maintained at 100–106°F before transporting.
d. Cover the frozen part tightly in wet occlusive dressings.

99. Signs and symptoms of radiation sickness include which of the following?
a. severe headache
b. excessive thirst
c. hair loss
d. hearing problems

100. Why would a paramedic give diphenhydramine (Benadryl) to a schizophrenic patient in the field?
a. to help control his or her manic symptoms
b. to help counteract catatonic symptoms
c. to raise blood pressure and respiratory rate
d. to counteract adverse medication reactions

101. Which of the following represents a significant mechanism of injury?
a. A small child is in a 40 mph car accident.
b. An adult falls from a 6-foot-high ledge.
c. An adult pedestrian is hit by a bicycle.
d. A child falls from a 4-foot-high ledge.

Answer questions 102–106 based on the following information.

You arrive to find a six-year-old boy on the floor of his classroom, unconscious, incontinent, and responsive to pain only. The school nurse states that the child shook violently for approximately two minutes and, following, has been unconscious. She knows that he takes phenobarbital because she gave him one at lunch, but she is unable to provide further medical history.

102. This child most likely suffers from which of the following?
a. diabetes mellitus
b. diabetes insipidus
c. seizure disorder
d. status asthmaticus

103. Phenobarbital is an example of which class or type of medication?
   a. synthetic form of insulin
   b. sedative or anticonvulsant
   c. hypoglycemic medication
   d. beta agonist agent

104. If this child is on medication, why did he have this episode at school?
   a. Medications only limit the number of seizures a person has; they do not always eliminate the seizures.
   b. Medication for this disorder does not control the amount of glucose available for cellular metabolism.
   c. This child may have had too much to eat, overriding the medication's ability to regulate blood sugar.
   d. The school nurse must have been mistaken in administering the medication to the child at lunch.

105. Treatment for this patient should include which of the following?
   a. 50% dextrose solution
   b. 25% dextrose solution
   c. diazepam (Valium)
   d. oxygen and monitoring

106. Why should this patient be transported to a hospital?
   a. He needs a lumbar puncture to determine if he has meningitis.
   b. Medication levels need to be determined by laboratory analysis.
   c. Glucose levels need to be determined by laboratory analysis.
   d. Repeat episodes will continue without hospitalization.

107. Which of the following is the ideal helicopter landing zone?
   a. an area with a slope of no more than 15°
   b. an area of at least 100 feet by 100 feet
   c. an area of at least 90 feet by 90 feet
   d. a fenced area for safety against onlookers

108. Your patient is ten months old. He has tachypnea and wheezing and a fever of 100.6°F. What do you suspect is wrong with your patient?
   a. asthma
   b. epiglottitis
   c. bronchiolitis
   d. croup

109. Cardiac arrest in young children is most commonly associated with which of the following?
   a. respiratory problems or diseases
   b. trauma from automobile accidents
   c. burn trauma from house fires
   d. underlying cardiac disease processes

110. Assessment and care of a patient who is a victim of sexual assault should include which of the following?
   a. Perform a complete vaginal exam.
   b. Ask detailed questions about the assault.
   c. Place sterile dressings on any wounds.
   d. Allow the patient to bathe and douche.

111. Which statement characterizes normal physiologic changes that occur in vital signs during pregnancy?
   a. blood pressure falls; pulse rate rises
   b. blood pressure falls; pulse rate falls
   c. blood pressure rises; pulse rate rises
   d. blood pressure rises; pulse rate falls

112. You are recording vital signs for a 34-year-old woman who is eight months pregnant. Her blood pressure is 100/70 mmHg, pulse rate is 80 BPM, and respirations are 17 breaths per minute and normal. Upon auscultation of her chest, you hear a mild systolic flow murmur. How should you treat this patient?
   a. Transport her immediately to a facility with OB/GYN services for her imminent delivery.
   b. Establish an IV, administer high-flow oxygen, and monitor vital signs every two minutes.
   c. The murmur is not a finding of concern; document these findings on the patient-care report.
   d. Continue to assess the patient for additional signs or symptoms of left-sided heart failure.

113. Your patient is a 29-year-old woman who is nine months pregnant with her third child. She reports the onset of painless, bright red vaginal bleeding in the past half hour. How should you treat this patient?
   a. Perform a vaginal exam to determine if this is a placental abruption.
   b. Check for crowning, perineal bulging, or other signs of impending delivery.
   c. Wait for delivery and then transport both mother and child to the hospital.
   d. Treat her for signs and symptoms of shock and transport immediately.

114. You are assessing a neonate who has a pink body and blue extremities, a pulse rate of 90, weak grimace response, active motion, and irregular respiratory efforts. What is the Apgar score for this infant?
   a. 4
   b. 6
   c. 8
   d. 10

115. Which of the following characteristics is the criterion for administering positive pressure ventilation to a newborn?
   a. Apnea was corrected with blow-by oxygen use.
   b. The heart rate rose from 90 to 110 in two minutes.
   c. Central cyanosis persists while oxygen is given.
   d. Meconium staining was noted during delivery.

Answer questions 116–118 based on the following information.

You respond to the home of a two-year-old girl who is experiencing labored and difficult breathing. The child's mother states that the child has had a cold for the past several days and a seal-like bark for the past 20 minutes. Physical exam reveals she has a fever of 102°F and hot, dry skin. Inspiratory stridor is heard upon auscultation of lung sounds. Vital signs are blood pressure of 100/70 mmHg, pulse rate of 100 BPM, and respiratory rate of 40 breaths per minute that is labored and with sternal retractions noted.

116. This patient is most likely suffering from which of the following?
   a. upper-airway obstruction
   b. epiglottitis
   c. aspiration pneumonia
   d. croup

117. What is the appropriate treatment for this child?
   a. examination of the oropharynx with a tongue blade
   b. direct visualization of the vocal cords for swelling
   c. nebulized albuterol and cooling measures en route
   d. saline given by nebulizer treatment and oxygen

118. A related disease or condition that can result in rapid and total airway obstruction is which of the following?
   a. bronchitis
   b. epiglottitis
   c. bronchiolitis
   d. laryngitis

119. A tiered response system is one that does which of the following?
   a. dispatches responders at various levels depending on the incident
   b. dispatches ALS responders to arrive first to all medical emergencies
   c. dispatches ALS responders on fire trucks instead of ambulances
   d. uses chase vehicles staffed with ALS providers to drive ambulances

120. A victim is unresponsive after possible exposure to carbon monoxide in a closed garage. Which of the following procedures should you do first?
   a. Wait for properly trained personnel to enter and evacuate the garage.
   b. Open the windows of the garage to ventilate the environment.
   c. Provide high-flow oxygen to the patient via positive pressure ventilations.
   d. Remove the patient from the environment.

121. With whom does ultimate responsibility for patient care in the field always rest?
   a. the highest trained provider on scene
   b. the regional or state EMS director
   c. the medical control physician
   d. whoever provides online direction

122. The rhythm that appears in the ECG shown in Figure 3.1 is which of the following?
   a. first-degree AV block
   b. second-degree AV block type I
   c. second-degree AV block type II
   d. third-degree AV block

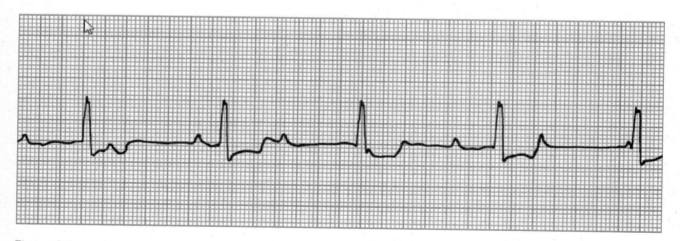

Figure 3.1

123. Which of the following situations represents expressed consent?
  a. The patient says, "Help me. My chest hurts."
  b. The patient is eight years old with no parent present.
  c. The patient is unconscious and unresponsive.
  d. The patient says, "I don't need any help. Just let me die."

124. An intoxicated person refuses treatment or transport. How should you proceed?
  a. Do as the patient wishes and leave the scene immediately.
  b. Try to find a family member to get consent for treatment.
  c. Try to persuade the person to accept your assistance.
  d. Immediately document the refusal, and then leave the scene.

125. Patients who have overdosed and have altered mental status are best transported in which position?
  a. supine
  b. prone
  c. left-lateral recumbent
  d. full Fowler's

126. What is the purpose of the START method?
  a. to coordinate the efforts of multiple response units to a mass casualty incident (MCI)
  b. to ensure safe access of responding units to the MCI site
  c. to rapidly triage large numbers of patients quickly and efficiently
  d. to communicate with medical personnel as efficiently as possible

127. What is the first step in triage at an MCI?
  a. direct the walking wounded away from the scene
  b. assess the victims' respiratory status and pulse rate
  c. assess the victims' hemodynamic status and AVPU
  d. valuate the victims' mental status and ABCs

128. What are the three primary parameters assessed when using the START triage system?
  a. airway, breathing, and circulation (ABC)
  b. respiration, perfusion, and mentation (RPM)
  c. appearance, respiration, and mentation (ARM)
  d. pulse, perfusion, and perspiration (PPP)

129. Which communications system has the capability to send and receive voice and telemetry simultaneously?
  a. VHF
  b. multiplex
  c. UHF
  d. duplex

130. Which of the following correctly describes pulsus paradoxus?
  a. an abnormal decrease in the systolic pressure during inspiration compared with expiration
  b. an abnormal increase in the systolic pressure during inspiration compared with expiration
  c. an abnormal decrease in pulse rate between the radial and carotid pulses during inspiration compared with expiration
  d. an abnormal increase in pulse rate between the radial and carotid pulses during inspiration compared with expiration

131. Ventilating a patient at 30 breaths per minute with a bag-valve mask and high-flow oxygen may result in which of the following?
a. an increase in intracranial pressure
b. a decrease in the normal serum blood pH
c. alkalizing the bloodstream
d. production of a tension pneumothorax

132. Which patient is most likely to require immediate transport?
a. 25-year-old male, fractured wrist
b. 45-year-old male, fractured pelvis
c. 38-year-old female, fractured tibia
d. 52-year-old female, fractured humerus

Answer questions 133 and 134 based on the following information.

You respond to a 25-patient mass casualty incident at a store. The 911 caller stated that she smelled something "funny" and then started to feel weak and nauseous. You are the second unit on the scene. The initial unit is nowhere to be seen and they do not answer their radios.

133. What should you determine first in this situation?
a. whether the other crew is treating patients inside and needs your help
b. whether this is a potential hazardous-materials incident in progress
c. whether the other crew has been overcome and needs your immediate assistance
d. whether you need more oxygen and supplies than your ambulance carries

134. After you are instructed by the hazardous materials team to begin treating decontaminated patients, you should perform which of the following?
a. Take universal precautions and wear protective equipment.
b. Begin your efforts with the least symptomatic patient first.
c. Get ready to treat the patients as you would at any other scene.
d. Thoroughly question the first patient for purposes of documentation.

135. For which of the following procedures is a gown most necessary?
a. emergency childbirth
b. drawing blood
c. suctioning the airway
d. cleaning instruments

136. Which of the following requires intermediate-level disinfection through the use of a solution of bleach and water?
a. routine housecleaning measures in your station and bunkroom
b. any items that have come into contact with mucous membranes
c. any instruments that were used in any invasive procedures
d. all items that have come into contact with intact skin

137. Which infection is transmitted through contact with blood or body secretions?
a. hepatitis A
b. hepatitis B
c. varicella
d. tuberculosis

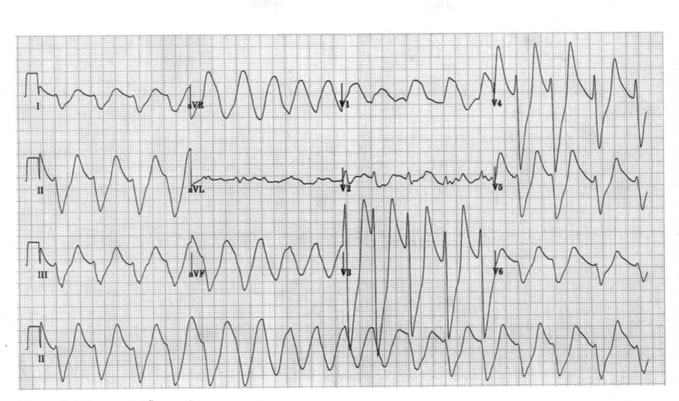

Figure 3.2 (www.pic2fly.com)

138. You have arrived on the scene to find a dialysis patient. The patient is responding to verbal stimuli with incomprehensible words. You can palpate a weak radial pulse and the patient is breathing 12 times per minute. Which of the following is an appropriate treatment for this patient? See Figure 3.2.
   a. synchronized cardioversion with 50 joules
   b. defibrillation at 150 joules
   c. administration of a 1.5 mg/kg lidocaine bolus IV
   d. administration of 1 g calcium chloride IV

139. Identify the rhythm depicted in Figure 3.3.
   a. ventricular fibrillation
   b. ventricular tachycardia
   c. supraventricular tachycardia
   d. PVC couplets

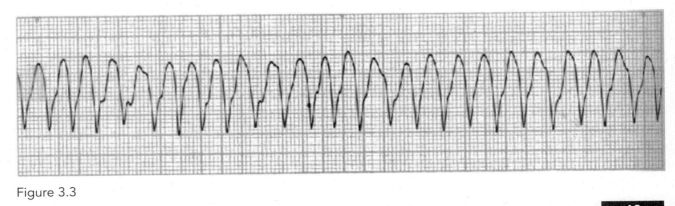

Figure 3.3

140. What anatomical structures and pathophysiology are most important for the paramedic to consider when determining the treatment of the airway of a patient who has suffered an inhalation burn injury?
   a. The cricoid cartilage, trachea, mainstem bronchus, and cilia within the lower airway
   b. The tonsils, uvula, epiglottis, larynx, and the vasculature of the upper airway
   c. The bronchioles, alveoli, and the surfactant of the lungs
   d. The nares, sinus cavities, and the mucous production in the sinuses

141. What is the purpose of the body's physiological response to a stressor?
   a. to signal the brain that danger is present
   b. to decrease normal physiological functions
   c. to shut down the autonomic nervous system
   d. to prepare for the most efficient reaction

142. Signs and symptoms of compensated shock in a child include which of the following?
   a. diaphoresis, tachypnea, tachycardia, hypotension, anxiety, and capillary refill greater than two seconds
   b. mechanism of injury indicative of significant injury, tachycardia, response only to painful stimuli, tachypnea, hypotension, capillary refill less than two seconds
   c. mechanism of injury indicative of significant injury, anxiety/irritability, tachycardia, and capillary refill greater than two seconds
   d. mechanism of injury indicative of significant injury, anxiety/irritability, tachycardia, capillary refill greater than two seconds, and hypotension

143. You respond to a call for a five-year-old male patient who has fallen 12 feet from a tree house. You would expect what type of injuries in this patient?
   a. forearm fractures
   b. head and neck injuries
   c. compression fractures of the lumbar spine
   d. sprains and dislocations of the ankle or knee

144. You respond to the local park for a ten-year-old male, who was tackled and landed on his left side. The patient states he landed on the football and complains of diffuse abdominal pain. Your exam reveals diffuse tenderness and voluntary guarding on palpation of the upper left quadrant. The patient's skin is cool and moist, and he is irritable and tachycardic. What injury is most likely causing your exam findings?
   a. lacerated liver
   b. ruptured stomach
   c. dissecting abdominal aortic aneurysm
   d. ruptured spleen

145. Identify the rhythm depicted in Figure 3.4.
   a. first-degree AV block
   b. second-degree AV block Mobitz type I
   c. normal sinus rhythm with PJCs
   d. second-degree AV block Mobitz type II

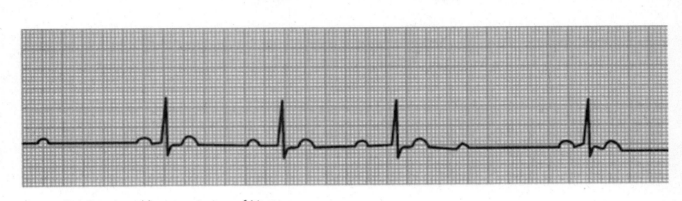

Figure 3.4 Reprinted by permission of Nott.

146. You are treating a 58-year-old female patient who complains of chest pain and dizziness. You have obtained an ECG that shows runs of ventricular tachycardia. You have administered two lidocaine boluses and she has converted to a sinus rhythm. Medical control has ordered a 2 mg/min. lidocaine drip. You have lidocaine premixed 100 mg in 250 mL of normal saline. Using a 60-drop administration set, how many drops per minute will you infuse?
   a. 48 drops/min.
   b. 75 drops/min.
   c. 120 drops/min.
   d. 300 drops/min.

147. Identify the rhythm in Figure 3.5.
   a. sinus arrest
   b. sinus rhythm
   c. sinus bradycardia
   d. sinus arrhythmia

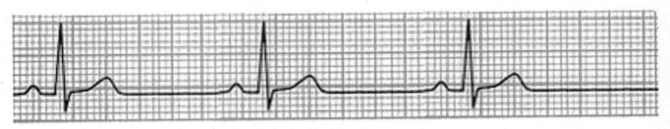

Figure 3.5 Reprinted by permission from Frank Conn (2004).

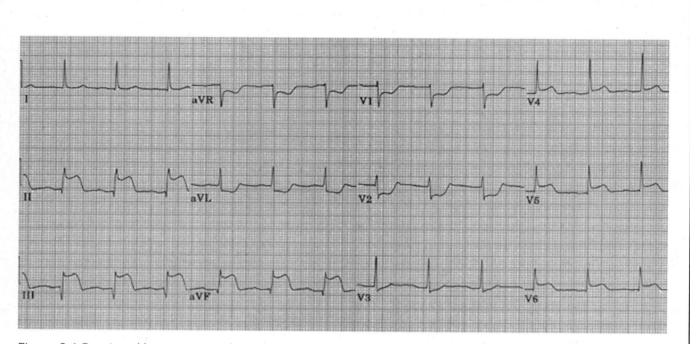

Figure 3.6 Reprinted by permission by Adam Szulewski.

148. Which of the following is the location of the infarct in the 12-lead ECG in Figure 3.6?
a. inferior wall MI
b. lateral wall MI
c. ECG is normal and not indicative of an MI
d. anteroseptal wall MI

149. Which of the following medications is a depolarizing paralytic agent?
a. etomidate
b. vecuronium
c. succinylcholine
d. rocuronium

150. Which of the following represents a normal tidal volume for an adult patient?
a. 1–5 mL/kg
b. 5–10 mL/kg
c. 10–15 mL/kg
d. 15–20 mL/kg

Answers

1. c. Both good stress (*eustress*) and bad stress (*distress*) will initially cause sympathetic stimulation, such as increased heart and respiratory rate, bronchodilation, dilated pupils, and increased blood flow to the skeletal muscles.

2. b. No carbon dioxide after six ventilations indicates either that the tube is in the esophagus or that the patient has been dead long enough that no carbon dioxide is being produced.

3. a. The purpose of the focused history and physical exam is to detect additional problems after you have controlled immediate threats to the patient's life. The ongoing assessment is typically performed during transport. Medical control may be consulted anytime during the call when you feel it is appropriate, or whenever your protocols and standing orders require medical control contact.

4. d. This patient is exhibiting the classic signs and symptoms of an abdominal aortic aneurysm (AAA). Further palpation may cause the aneurysm to rupture, so be very careful in assessing this patient. The other choices will not cause abdominal pulsations to occur.

5. a. Cardiac monitoring should always be performed when you suspect that an aneurysm is present. Rapid infusion of crystalloid solution is often indicated in the treatment of shock, but the fluid must be titrated to patient response. Dopamine is indicated for cardiogenic shock. Shock in this patient would be due to hypovolemia. Dopamine is contraindicated in the presence of uncorrected hypovolemia. PASG/MAST may be indicated for treatment of AAA in some jurisdictions; however, it is not a standardized treatment.

6. a. Chronic obstructive pulmonary disease (COPD) patients can no longer rely up normal regulatory mechanisms to control their respirations. The hypoxic drive measures for low levels of oxygen in the bloodstream to increase respiratory rate.

7. b. The posterior tibial pulse is assessed just below and posterior to where the ankle bone protrudes medially. The pulse located on the top of the foot is the dorsalis pedis. The popliteal pulse is located behind the knee.

8. b. Cheyne-Stokes respirations are characterized by an increase in rate and depth followed by a gradual decrease in rate and depth and intermittent periods of apnea. Agonal respirations are an irregular, gasping, slow, and shallow pattern of respiration. Kussmaul respirations appear as deep, rapid, and regular respirations. Biot's breathing is an irregular pattern, rate, and depth with periods of apnea.

9. a. Indications for immediate transport include any signs or symptoms of shock: sustained pulse rate greater than 120 BPM or less than 50 BPM, systolic BP less than 90 mmHg, and respiratory rate less than ten breaths per minute or greater than 29 breaths per minute. Based only on these vital signs, the first patient appears already to be in shock.

10. b. This change in vital signs comprises Cushing's reflex, a sign of increasing intracranial pressure. Cushing's reflex is also sometimes called Cushing's triad or Cushing's response.

11. c. The most appropriate dressing for an evisceration is the application of a wet sterile dressing (which keeps the organs moist) and an occlusive dressing (which provides a barrier against further contamination and heat loss).

12. d. Each fracture has a potential blood loss of one or more units per fracture site. Because of its ring shape, the pelvis frequently has two or more fractures present. In addition, nerve and blood vessel damage and genitourinary organ injuries can complicate the severity of this injury. Patients with pelvis fractures are always considered high-priority patients and should be rapidly stabilized and transported. If a patient has bilateral femur fractures, he or she is also a high-priority patient.

13. d. A unilaterally dilated pupil may be an early sign of increased intracranial pressure. As swelling increases in the brain, it puts pressure on the optic nerve that is located near the area of swelling.

14. a. The technique of palpation uses touch during a physical examination to gather information. Percussion is using gentle tapping in order to identify the presence of air or fluid in body tissues. Palpitations are heartbeat sensations that feel like your heart is pounding or racing. Auscultation is listening with a stethoscope.

15. a. Stridor can usually be heard without a stethoscope and emanates from the area of the throat.

16. b. Choices **a**, **c**, and **d** all indicate *some* air exchange.

17. a. The other three choices, while serious, generally would not cause an absence of breath sounds.

18. c. The bridge of the nose in a pediatric patient may make a mask seal more difficult to achieve. Additionally, the mask size needed to fit the pediatric patient's face may not be available.

19. c. If the patient is unconscious and vomits, the PTL will help prevent aspiration. Instead, if a gag reflex returns, the PTL will have to be removed before the patient vomits.

20. a. Medical patients who are stable should be in a position of comfort.

21. c. Use only gentle palpation in the field. Correctly performed percussion requires a relatively quiet environment and an experienced hand to be of any diagnostic value. Properly performed auscultation for bowel sounds takes several minutes and is of little value to your overall treatment regimen. Continued assessment for rebound tenderness will aggravate the patient's discomfort and is unnecessary once you have determined that the patient has abdominal distress.

22. b. The dosage of many common medications is up to 50% lower in elderly adults primarily because of a decreased rate of elimination of the drug by the liver and kidneys.

23. c. A patient with left heart failure will present with elevated blood pressure, elevated and sometimes irregular pulse, and labored respirations.

24. c. $PaCO_2$ measures carbon dioxide levels in the blood, which are influenced by alterations in CO_2 production or elimination. Such levels would be increased by physical exertion of muscles, by hypoventilation, or by an airway obstruction.

25. a. Tidal volume is the amount of air that moves into or out of the lungs during the respiratory cycle. Total lung capacity is the sum of the inspiratory reserve, tidal volume, expiratory reserve, and residual volume. Minute volume is the amount of air that moves in and out of the lungs in one minute. Inspiratory reserve is the extra air that could be inspired in addition to the tidal volume.

26. c. The vital signs given in this choice are most likely for a patient with CHF who is complaining of difficulty breathing.

27. d. Diuretics, potassium, and digoxin are the common medications used to treat CHF.

28. b. The pulmonary edema associated with CHF commonly results in crackles and/or rhonchi, especially in the lower lobes.

29. a. CHF results from the cardiac muscle's inability to pump efficiently.

30. c. Excessive pressure against the delicate soft tissue of the lower airway may reduce blood flow to the site, causing ischemia.

31. a. To ensure proper placement, always confirm by at least two different methods. After watching the tube pass through the vocal cords, assess the chest for breath sounds in numerous locations and chest expansion, and then check the proximal end of the tube for breath condensation. You may also use one of several commercial confirmation devices that monitor end-tidal CO_2 using litmus paper or continuous waveform capnography.

32. a. The *T* in DCAP-BTLS stands for tenderness.

33. c. Excessive pressure inside the thoracic cavity due to the tension pneumothorax will result in all of the described signs.

34. a. Attempts at suctioning should be limited to no more than five to ten seconds (depending on the level of consciousness). You should ventilate the patient after each attempt, and you should not turn on the apparatus until the catheter is placed properly. If a suction catheter has a hole in the system that allows you to control suction by occluding the opening, you should only suction upon withdrawal. This system may remain turned on at all times as long as you monitor closely when suction is actually being applied to the patient.

35. a. The signs and symptoms listed describe a tension pneumothorax—the presence of air in the pleural space and mediastinal shifting.

36. a. Dyspnea, crackles, and rhonchi are classic signs of fluid overload, which is usually first manifested as pulmonary edema.

37. a. For the conscious patient, your first action would be abdominal thrusts.

38. c. Low-flow oxygen is appropriate for this patient if he or she is not hypoxic. If a patient with emphysema or chronic bronchitis is hypoxic, he or she needs more oxygen.

39. c. Albuterol, a bronchodilator sold under the trade names Proventil and Ventolin, is frequently given via inhaler or nebulizer in the field.

40. d. Place your hand on the patient's wrist as if you were measuring his or her pulse and count for 30 seconds. This will prevent the patient from consciously changing the respiratory rate. Placing the wrist and hand over the patient's chest wall is called the *pledge of allegiance* method.

41. d. According to AHA standards regarding a conscious patient with a partially obstructed airway, you should encourage coughing and continuously monitor the patient's status. Interventions like the Heimlich maneuver are considered counterproductive, as they may actually worsen the obstruction.

42. d. A hyperextended position will place the anatomical structures into a position that can be easily identified by palpation.

43. a. A patient in respiratory distress is compensating for the underlying condition, thereby preserving oxygenation to the brain. Once compensatory mechanisms have failed, the loss of gas exchange in the brain will result in a change in mental status.

44. a. Hyperextending the neck of a small child may result in an unintentional closure of the airway due to the softer cartilage rings supporting the trachea.

45. c. Cheyne-Stokes respirations are characterized by periods of apnea lasting 10–60 seconds, followed by periods in which respirations gradually increase, then decrease, in depth and rate.

46. b. Because seawater is hypertonic, fluid is drawn from the bloodstream into the alveoli, causing pulmonary edema. Because of this, all drowning (in seawater) patients should be hospitalized and monitored for a short time.

47. c. This victim of smoke inhalation is exhibiting the classic signs and symptoms of carbon monoxide poisoning.

48. a. This is a common finding with the use of pulse oximetry in carbon monoxide poisoning. The CO molecule, which has a high affinity for hemoglobin, is bound to the molecule and is present for detection as "oxygen" in blood passing through the capillary beds, resulting in fairly normal pulse oximetry readings. However, little, if any, of the oxygen is off-loaded from the hemoglobin molecule for use by the tissues.

49. c. If a hyperbaric chamber is available, this patient should be transported there immediately. Hyperbaric oxygen can dramatically improve outcomes for CO poisoning by reducing the time it takes for the CO molecule to unbind from the hemoglobin molecule. Low-flow oxygen and sodium bicarbonate are not indicated for carbon monoxide poisoning. The patient is unconscious, so position of comfort is not an issue. If you suspect the possibility of a spinal injury, you should immobilize this patient to a long backboard.

50. d. Hyperactivity is not a sign of carbon monoxide exposure. Generally, patients are lethargic due to being hypoxic.

51. a. Engine exhaust is a common source of carbon monoxide. Improperly ventilated space heaters are another source. Cellular metabolism and cellular respiration result in the formation of carbon dioxide.

52. c. Because the patient appears fatigued, respiratory failure is imminent. Inadequate tidal volume may not permit good gas exchange without manual support.

53. d. To manage acute anaphylaxis, you should first use epinephrine, followed by diphenhydramine. Epinephrine is a potent antihistamine and immediately reverses the physiological effects of the reaction (vasodilation, bronchoconstriction, and airway swelling), while diphenhydramine slows and stops the reaction itself.

54. b. Proper flow cannot be achieved if the constricting band (tourniquet) is not removed.

55. c. Indications for use of the PASG are to control bleeding, stabilize fractures, and raise blood pressure. Although its use is currently controversial, of the choices listed, choice **c** has the indications called for if PASG is to be used.

56. d. Patients with cardiac contusion can present with the symptoms of myocardial infarction, including life-threatening dysrhythmias. Care is similar to care of any cardiac patient.

57. d. The loss of lingual control during unconsciousness occurs more commonly than the other conditions.

58. a. In the down-and-under pathway, the body slides forward and downward. The up-and-over pathway refers to injuries sustained in the head, neck, and chest region. This can be limited by the correct use of seat belts.

59. b. The QRS complex reflects the underlying ventricular depolarization; buried within it is the atrial repolarization.

60. a. If the patient is asymptomatic, this arrhythmia requires observation only. Other treatments described are for patients with varying degrees of supraventricular tachycardia.

61. d. Ligamentum arteriosum is the most common area for an aortic rupture secondary to trauma.

62. d. First-degree AV block in itself calls for observation only; however, it may indicate the development of a more advanced heart block.

63. a. When stress or excessive caffeine intake in a patient with no history of heart disease causes PJT, the Valsalva maneuver can be successful at slowing the heart rate.

64. c. Because the underlying cause is usually ischemia, an accelerated junctional rhythm can deteriorate into more serious dysrhythmias.

65. d. Check for jugular vein distention with the patient elevated at a 45° angle. Most patients will have observable jugular veins when supine.

66. b. A bruit, noisy blood flow in a vessel, indicates partial obstruction due to plaque buildup or the presence of an embolus.

67. a. A strong force striking the car from behind causes the head to move backward. If the head restraint is not properly placed, it can actually act as a fulcrum, causing the neck to hyperextend. Then the head snaps forward, with the chin pointing toward the chest. This results in a severe hyperflexion of the neck.

68. a. Attacks of stable angina are brought on by exercise or by stress and are usually easily managed.

69. a. These are classic signs and symptoms of left heart failure with pulmonary edema.

70. c. Right heart failure, unless it is accompanied by left heart failure with pulmonary edema, is not a true medical emergency and does not require rapid transport.

71. b. Lidocaine is a first-line drug in the treatment of dysrhythmias.

72. b. Emergency synchronized cardioversion is synchronized with the R wave in order to avoid firing during the relative refractory period, which could induce ventricular tachycardia.

73. b. The correct protocol for stable angina is rest, oxygen, and nitroglycerin.

74. a. The wheezing, due to bronchoconstriction of smooth muscle in the lung, is a reaction to fluid in the lung spaces.

75. d. Flat neck veins while the patient is supine indicate a lower than normal pressure inside the vasculature, most likely due to blood loss. This would indicate a hemothorax as the primary cause of the described signs and symptoms.

76. b. Diazepam given through the IM route is ineffective. Nasal intubation may raise intracranial pressure even higher. Oral intubation may be difficult to achieve through clenched teeth.

77. d. A too-rapid ascent from a scuba dive may result in a pulmonary embolism due to lung overinflation.

78. b. An IV, 100% oxygen via a nonrebreather mask, and transport to a recompression chamber are essential for this patient.

79. c. Due to the depth of the dive and the rapid ascent, this patient may also be suffering from decompression sickness.

80. b. In this patient, nitrogen gas bubbles may have entered tissue spaces and blood vessels.

81. d. Intravenous thiamine is used to reverse the effects of acute thiamine deficiency, which may lead to seizures and encephalopathy in alcoholics.

82. a. Suction the newborn before stimulating it to breathe. Endotracheal suctioning may be warranted if meconium is noted in the upper airway.

83. c. A greenstick fracture is a partial fracture that is on only one side of the long bone. These fractures are noted most frequently in children but may also be seen in adults.

84. a. This is the current field treatment regimen for pelvic fractures. Patients with a suspected pelvic fracture should have a pelvic wrap applied to close the pelvis. If a pelvic wrap is unavailable, PASG/MAST can be used.

85. d. The correct treatment for powder or solid chemical burns is to first brush off as much of the chemical as possible and then flush with cool water and continue throughout transport.

86. d. The first step in managing a burn is to stop the burning process or the burn will continue to destroy more tissue. Then attention should turn toward ensuring and maintaining an adequate airway.

87. b. Blister formation is characteristic of second-degree burns.

88. c. Using the rule of nines, this patient has burns over 27% of her body surface area (both sides of one arm = 9%; both sides of one leg = 18%).

89. a. This patient is showing signs and symptoms of diabetic ketoacidosis. Avoid the use of glucose administration if at all possible. At the minimum, you should obtain a glucometer reading before administering any glucose-containing solutions. The fluid bolus will help dilute the glucose contained within his blood.

90. b. These are the classic signs of hypoglycemia.

91. a. Naloxone (Narcan) is a narcotic antagonist given to patients suspected of narcotic ingestion.

92. b. Major decontamination and treatment for life-threatening conditions should be conducted by properly protected personnel in the warm zone.

93. b. Epinephrine is the first-line drug for patients with severe allergic reactions. Oxygen, albuterol, and terbutaline are all respiratory drugs, but they do not have any antihistamine properties. Diphenhydramine (Benadryl) is an antihistamine and will stop the production of histamine, the chemical responsible for the exaggerated immune response.

94. d. Beta agonists such as albuterol help in the treatment of severe allergic reactions by relaxing the airway and thus relieving bronchospasm.

95. c. Alpha particles carry very little energy. A cloth uniform is adequate protection against such a contaminant.

96. a. The symptoms of organophosphate absorption are described by the acronym SLUDGE: (excessive) salivation, lacrimation, urination, diarrhea, gastrointestinal distress, emesis.

97. b. Moderate hypothermia is characterized by a core temperature between 86°F and 94°F.

98. a. The correct treatment is gradual warming in a water bath maintained between 100°F and 106°F, although this treatment should not be attempted in the field because of the danger of refreezing. Pain management is essential because the procedure is extremely painful.

99. c. Hair loss, nausea, and vomiting are common signs and symptoms of radiation sickness.

100. d. Benadryl is used to counter extrapyramidal reactions in patients who are taking antipsychotic drugs. Effects noted are involuntary movement, changes in muscle tone, and abnormal posture.

101. a. A 40 mph car accident is a significant mechanism of injury for a child but not for an adult unless there are other significant findings (lack of seat belts or another person is killed in the same car).

102. c. The clinical presentation of seizures could occur for a variety of reasons, including diabetes. However, the use of the drug phenobarbital is commonly associated with seizure disorders.

103. b. Phenobarbital is a sedative or anticonvulsant.

104. a. Anticonvulsants serve to limit the number of seizures a patient has, but they do not stop them from occurring altogether.

105. d. The medications listed in choices **a**, **b**, and **c** are not indicated for postictal patients who have stopped seizing.

106. b. This patient needs to be transported to a hospital so that medication levels can be assessed by laboratory methods. Seizures may or may not continue to occur.

107. b. The ideal helicopter landing zone should be at least 100 feet by 100 feet square. Larger helicopters may require more room, so consult local air medical services if you are unsure of the size of aircraft used in your area. The ground slope should be no more than 10° and the area should be clear of debris, fences, wires, or other obstructions.

108. c. Epiglottitis will often have a fever higher than 100.6°F, and the epiglottitis patient will be drooling as respiratory distress worsens. Asthma in children this young often presents as coughing. Wheezing and tachypnea in a child younger than age 1 are most often due to bronchiolitis brought on by the RSV virus. Croup will present with junky-sounding airways and the classic seal-barking cough.

109. a. Most childhood cardiac arrests are the result of preventable accidents that result in respiratory compromise.

110. c. Do not perform a vaginal exam, ask detailed questions about the assault in the field, or allow the patient to change clothes or bathe. You should not overly clean any wounds you encounter, but instead wrap them up with dry sterile dressings. Place any clothing or other evidence removed from the patient in a clean paper bag and take it with you to the hospital.

111. a. During pregnancy, a woman's blood pressure usually falls during the first two trimesters and her pulse rate rises.

112. c. A mild systolic murmur in a pregnant patient whose vital signs are normal is not a cause for concern.

113. d. Bright red bleeding in late pregnancy is assumed to be placenta previa, which is a true medical emergency that is life threatening to both mother and baby. Treat the mother for shock and transport immediately.

114. b. The score would consist of one point each for appearance, pulse rate, grimace, and respiratory effort, and two points for activity.

115. c. Apnea and tachycardia may initially be present in the newborn, but once they are corrected, you do not need to continue to progress further into the inverted pyramid. Meconium staining is treated first with suction. The child may or may not require ventilator support once it is cleared away.

116. d. This patient is exhibiting the classic signs and symptoms of croup.

117. d. A nebulized saline mist is the appropriate treatment for croup. Do not interfere with the airway in case there is any tissue swelling present.

118. b. Epiglottitis, a condition whereby the patient's airway can become totally obstructed, is related to croup.

119. a. In a tiered system, responders are dispatched to calls depending on the nature of the incident as stated by the 911 caller and evaluated by the dispatcher.

120. a. Safety first! Of the three extrication options, properly trained and protected rescuers can remove the patient safely.

121. c. No matter who is actually providing care or giving directions to the responder, ultimate responsibility always rests with the medical control physician.

122. d. The rhythm identified in Figure 3.1 is third-degree AV block.

123. a. Expressed consent means that the patient gives you permission to treat him or her, either verbally or in writing.

124. c. If a person who needs help refuses to accept it, you should try to persuade the person to accept aid and explain the consequences of refusing it. If the intoxicated patient continues to refuse, contact local law enforcement and medical control for assistance.

125. c. There is significant opportunity for the loss of airway control for this patient. A lateral recumbent position will allow passive draining of the airway in case of vomiting, as well as easy access for suctioning.

126. c. START stands for Simple Triage and Rapid Treatment and is designed to triage large numbers of patients as quickly as possible.

127. a. Regardless of the triage method utilized, the first step is to direct the walking wounded to a safe place where they can be cared for and reassessed.

128. b. Using the START triage system, the three primary parameters assessed are respiration, perfusion, and mentation (RPM). The parameters are a respiratory rate over or under 30 per minute, capillary refill under or over two seconds or presence of a radial pulse, and mentation (e.g., whether the patient is able to follow basic commands).

129. b. Duplex can send and receive voice only. UHF and VHF are bandwidth frequencies.

130. a. Pulsus paradoxus is an abnormal decrease in systolic blood pressure that drops more than 10 to 15 mmHg during inspiration compared with expiration. Normally, the systolic pressure decreases 5 to 10 mmHg during inspiration. However, in patients with asthma, COPD, pericardial tamponade, pulmonary embolism, or tension pneumothorax, the systolic pressure may decrease 10 to 20 mmHg or more during inspiration.

131. c. Hyperventilation may result in respiratory alkalosis, a harmful condition to the patient.

132. b. Because of the possibility of severe blood loss, patients with fractures of the pelvis are most likely to need immediate transport.

133. b. This is a hazardous-materials incident until proven otherwise. Do not rush in after fallen rescuers, because you may become a victim, too.

134. a. Always wear personal protective equipment to help avoid becoming contaminated. Unless you are trained to work in the hot zone, you should not treat anyone until they are properly decontaminated.

135. a. Wearing a gown is considered part of your body substance isolation (BSI) precautions with emergency childbirth. It may be recommended in some circumstances when cleaning instruments or drawing blood, but is not generally needed.

136. d. All instruments and supplies that have come into contact with intact skin require intermediate-level disinfection.

137. b. Hepatitis B is a blood-borne disease that is transmitted through contact with blood or body secretions.

138. d. The rhythm is a classic sine wave that can be mistaken for ventricular tachycardia. The patient's presentation gives you the clues that this is a sine wave most likely caused by hyperkalemia and not ventricular tachycardia with a pulse. The correct treatment for this patient is the administration of calcium chloride IV push. Follow local protocols for the appropriate dosage.

139. b. The rhythm indicates ventricular tachycardia.

140. b. The structures of the upper airway are responsible for the warming, cooling, and humidifying of inhaled air. The vascular nature of these structures makes them most susceptible to injury from an inhalation burn.

141. d. All the components of the stress reaction—release of ACTH, relaxation of the bronchial tree, slowdown of digestion, release of adrenaline—prepare the body to react to the stressor as efficiently as possible.

142. c. Compensated shock should be assumed and treated in any pediatric patient with a mechanism of injury suggesting serious injury and even subtle changes in mental status or perfusion status. Children compensate for blood loss very well and maintain their blood pressure until late in the decompensated phase.

143. b. Young children who fall from a height tend to land head first, therefore suffering head and neck injuries. Adults tend to land feet first and suffer leg and lumbar spine compression injuries.

144. d. The spleen is located in the upper left quadrant of the abdomen and is often injured in falls and sports-related injuries.

145. b. The progressively lengthening P-R interval and then a dropped QRS are indicative of a second-degree AV block Mobitz type I. First-degree blocks involve a lengthened P-R interval, but each P-R interval is the same. Second-degree AV block Mobitz type II is indicated by a constant P-R interval and a dropped QRS.

146. d. You have 100 mg in 250 mL of normal saline, which is a concentration of 0.4 mg/mL. You are using a 60-drop set, which gives you 60 drops/mL; therefore, the rate is 0.4 mg/RO. To get 2 mg/min. you need to infuse 300 drops per minute.

147. c. This strip indicates sinus bradycardia: the ECG is normal, but the rate is less than 60 beats per minute.

148. a. This 12-lead ECG reveals ST elevation in lead II, III, and AVF, which is indicative of an inferior wall MI.

149. c. Succinylcholine is the only depolarizing paralytic agent currently used. Etomidate is not a paralytic agent, and vecuronium and rocuronium are both nondepolarizing paralytic agents.

150. b. Normal adult tidal volume is 5–10 mL/kg.

Scoring

Evaluate how you did on this practice exam by first finding the number of questions you got right. Only the number of correct answers is important—questions you skipped or got wrong don't count against your score. Your goal should be a score greater than 80%. The NREMT exam is now computer adaptive and therefore there is no minimum score, just a measure of competency.

Use your scores in conjunction with the LearningExpress Test Preparation System in Chapter 2 of this book to help devise a study plan. You should plan to spend more time on the topics that correspond to the questions you found hardest, and less time on the lessons that correspond to areas in which you did well.

Much more important than your overall score, for now, is how you did on each of the topics tested by the exam. You need to diagnose your strengths and weaknesses so that you can concentrate your efforts as you prepare. The question types are mixed in the practice exam, so in order to tell where your strengths and weaknesses lie, you will need to compare your answer sheet with the following table, which shows the topics for each question.

PARAMEDIC PRACTICE EXAM 1 DIAGNOSTIC SCORING CHART	
TOPIC	QUESTION #
Airway, Respiration, and Ventilation	2, 6, 8, 15, 16, 17, 18, 19, 24, 25, 30, 31, 34, 37, 38, 39, 40, 41, 42, 43, 44, 45, 52, 57, 94, 116, 117, 118, 131, 149, 150
Cardiology and Resuscitation	23, 26, 27, 28, 29, 59, 60, 62, 63, 64, 66, 68, 69, 70, 71, 72, 73, 74, 109, 122, 138, 139, 145, 146, 147, 148
Trauma	7, 9, 10, 11, 12, 13, 32, 33, 35, 55, 56, 58, 61, 67, 75, 76, 83, 84, 85, 86, 87, 88, 101, 132, 140, 142, 143, 144
Medical/Obstetrics/ Gynecology	1, 3, 4, 5, 20, 21, 22, 46, 47, 48, 49, 50, 51, 53, 77, 78, 79, 80, 81, 82, 89, 90, 91, 93, 96, 97, 98, 99, 100, 102, 105, 106, 108, 111, 112, 113, 114, 115, 125, 130, 141
EMS Operations	14, 36, 54, 65, 92, 95, 103, 104, 107, 110, 119, 120, 121, 123, 124, 126, 127, 128, 129, 133, 134, 135, 136, 137

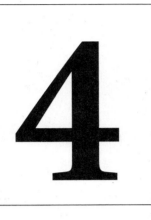

4 ▶ PARAMEDIC PRACTICE EXAM 2

CHAPTER SUMMARY

This is the second of five practice exams in this book based on the Paramedic written exam. Having taken one exam already, you should feel more confident in your ability to pick the correct answers. Use this exam to see how knowing what to expect makes you feel more prepared.

Like the first exam in this book, this exam is based on the official NREMT. It should not, however, feel precisely like the first test because now you know more about how the test is put together. You have seen how different types of questions are presented and should notice patterns in the order of questions. Questions on each area are grouped together. This pattern will help you develop your own test-taking strategy.

If you are following the advice of this book, you have studied between the first exam and this one. This second exam will give you a chance to see how much you have improved. We recommend that you study again following the grading of this exam as well. Do not concentrate your efforts only on the material in which you are weak. Factually dense material such as that on the NREMT EMT-Paramedic/ Paramedic exam calls for comprehensive reinforcement.

For this second exam, pay attention to the different types of questions and the relationship between questions on the same topic. (Also, you might want to try timing yourself to get an idea of the time needed to complete the actual exam.) Pay attention to the answer explanations, especially for the questions you missed.

1.	(a)	(b)	(c)	(d)	51.	(a)	(b)	(c)	(d)	101.	(a)	(b)	(c)	(d)
2.	(a)	(b)	(c)	(d)	52.	(a)	(b)	(c)	(d)	102.	(a)	(b)	(c)	(d)
3.	(a)	(b)	(c)	(d)	53.	(a)	(b)	(c)	(d)	103.	(a)	(b)	(c)	(d)
4.	(a)	(b)	(c)	(d)	54.	(a)	(b)	(c)	(d)	104.	(a)	(b)	(c)	(d)
5.	(a)	(b)	(c)	(d)	55.	(a)	(b)	(c)	(d)	105.	(a)	(b)	(c)	(d)
6.	(a)	(b)	(c)	(d)	56.	(a)	(b)	(c)	(d)	106.	(a)	(b)	(c)	(d)
7.	(a)	(b)	(c)	(d)	57.	(a)	(b)	(c)	(d)	107.	(a)	(b)	(c)	(d)
8.	(a)	(b)	(c)	(d)	58.	(a)	(b)	(c)	(d)	108.	(a)	(b)	(c)	(d)
9.	(a)	(b)	(c)	(d)	59.	(a)	(b)	(c)	(d)	109.	(a)	(b)	(c)	(d)
10.	(a)	(b)	(c)	(d)	60.	(a)	(b)	(c)	(d)	110.	(a)	(b)	(c)	(d)
11.	(a)	(b)	(c)	(d)	61.	(a)	(b)	(c)	(d)	111.	(a)	(b)	(c)	(d)
12.	(a)	(b)	(c)	(d)	62.	(a)	(b)	(c)	(d)	112.	(a)	(b)	(c)	(d)
13.	(a)	(b)	(c)	(d)	63.	(a)	(b)	(c)	(d)	113.	(a)	(b)	(c)	(d)
14.	(a)	(b)	(c)	(d)	64.	(a)	(b)	(c)	(d)	114.	(a)	(b)	(c)	(d)
15.	(a)	(b)	(c)	(d)	65.	(a)	(b)	(c)	(d)	115.	(a)	(b)	(c)	(d)
16.	(a)	(b)	(c)	(d)	66.	(a)	(b)	(c)	(d)	116.	(a)	(b)	(c)	(d)
17.	(a)	(b)	(c)	(d)	67.	(a)	(b)	(c)	(d)	117.	(a)	(b)	(c)	(d)
18.	(a)	(b)	(c)	(d)	68.	(a)	(b)	(c)	(d)	118.	(a)	(b)	(c)	(d)
19.	(a)	(b)	(c)	(d)	69.	(a)	(b)	(c)	(d)	119.	(a)	(b)	(c)	(d)
20.	(a)	(b)	(c)	(d)	70.	(a)	(b)	(c)	(d)	120.	(a)	(b)	(c)	(d)
21.	(a)	(b)	(c)	(d)	71.	(a)	(b)	(c)	(d)	121.	(a)	(b)	(c)	(d)
22.	(a)	(b)	(c)	(d)	72.	(a)	(b)	(c)	(d)	122.	(a)	(b)	(c)	(d)
23.	(a)	(b)	(c)	(d)	73.	(a)	(b)	(c)	(d)	123.	(a)	(b)	(c)	(d)
24.	(a)	(b)	(c)	(d)	74.	(a)	(b)	(c)	(d)	124.	(a)	(b)	(c)	(d)
25.	(a)	(b)	(c)	(d)	75.	(a)	(b)	(c)	(d)	125.	(a)	(b)	(c)	(d)
26.	(a)	(b)	(c)	(d)	76.	(a)	(b)	(c)	(d)	126.	(a)	(b)	(c)	(d)
27.	(a)	(b)	(c)	(d)	77.	(a)	(b)	(c)	(d)	127.	(a)	(b)	(c)	(d)
28.	(a)	(b)	(c)	(d)	78.	(a)	(b)	(c)	(d)	128.	(a)	(b)	(c)	(d)
29.	(a)	(b)	(c)	(d)	79.	(a)	(b)	(c)	(d)	129.	(a)	(b)	(c)	(d)
30.	(a)	(b)	(c)	(d)	80.	(a)	(b)	(c)	(d)	130.	(a)	(b)	(c)	(d)
31.	(a)	(b)	(c)	(d)	81.	(a)	(b)	(c)	(d)	131.	(a)	(b)	(c)	(d)
32.	(a)	(b)	(c)	(d)	82.	(a)	(b)	(c)	(d)	132.	(a)	(b)	(c)	(d)
33.	(a)	(b)	(c)	(d)	83.	(a)	(b)	(c)	(d)	133.	(a)	(b)	(c)	(d)
34.	(a)	(b)	(c)	(d)	84.	(a)	(b)	(c)	(d)	134.	(a)	(b)	(c)	(d)
35.	(a)	(b)	(c)	(d)	85.	(a)	(b)	(c)	(d)	135.	(a)	(b)	(c)	(d)
36.	(a)	(b)	(c)	(d)	86.	(a)	(b)	(c)	(d)	136.	(a)	(b)	(c)	(d)
37.	(a)	(b)	(c)	(d)	87.	(a)	(b)	(c)	(d)	137.	(a)	(b)	(c)	(d)
38.	(a)	(b)	(c)	(d)	88.	(a)	(b)	(c)	(d)	138.	(a)	(b)	(c)	(d)
39.	(a)	(b)	(c)	(d)	89.	(a)	(b)	(c)	(d)	139.	(a)	(b)	(c)	(d)
40.	(a)	(b)	(c)	(d)	90.	(a)	(b)	(c)	(d)	140.	(a)	(b)	(c)	(d)
41.	(a)	(b)	(c)	(d)	91.	(a)	(b)	(c)	(d)	141.	(a)	(b)	(c)	(d)
42.	(a)	(b)	(c)	(d)	92.	(a)	(b)	(c)	(d)	142.	(a)	(b)	(c)	(d)
43.	(a)	(b)	(c)	(d)	93.	(a)	(b)	(c)	(d)	143.	(a)	(b)	(c)	(d)
44.	(a)	(b)	(c)	(d)	94.	(a)	(b)	(c)	(d)	144.	(a)	(b)	(c)	(d)
45.	(a)	(b)	(c)	(d)	95.	(a)	(b)	(c)	(d)	145.	(a)	(b)	(c)	(d)
46.	(a)	(b)	(c)	(d)	96.	(a)	(b)	(c)	(d)	146.	(a)	(b)	(c)	(d)
47.	(a)	(b)	(c)	(d)	97.	(a)	(b)	(c)	(d)	147.	(a)	(b)	(c)	(d)
48.	(a)	(b)	(c)	(d)	98.	(a)	(b)	(c)	(d)	148.	(a)	(b)	(c)	(d)
49.	(a)	(b)	(c)	(d)	99.	(a)	(b)	(c)	(d)	149.	(a)	(b)	(c)	(d)
50.	(a)	(b)	(c)	(d)	100.	(a)	(b)	(c)	(d)	150.	(a)	(b)	(c)	(d)

Paramedic Exam 2

1. Your patient is a 27-year-old male who has fallen from a 24-foot ladder. As you are approaching and forming your general impression, you note that he is conscious and talking. What should you do first?
   a. Look at his chest to begin assessing the airway.
   b. Manually stabilize his neck in a neutral position.
   c. Palpate for a radial pulse in an uninjured arm.
   d. Palpate for a carotid pulse on one side of his neck.

2. You note snoring sounds during your initial assessment of a trauma patient who is responding to painful stimuli. What is your next step?
   a. Manually stabilize the cervical spine.
   b. Perform the jaw-thrust/chin-lift maneuver.
   c. Perform the head-tilt/chin-lift maneuver.
   d. Measure and insert an oropharyngeal airway.

3. With the START method, several vital signs are quickly assessed to determine the order to care for and transport patients. According to the START method, which of the following patients would receive immediate treatment to support hemodynamic status without further assessment?
   a. male, radial pulse present, skin warm and dry
   b. female, radial pulse present, capillary refill time of one sec
   c. male, radial pulse present, skin pale, and cyanotic
   d. female, radial pulse present, capillary refill time of 0.5 sec

4. A patient in compensatory hemorrhagic shock would most likely present with which set of vital signs?
   a. P 120 BPM and BP 122/86 mmHg
   b. P 80 BPM and BP 118/70 mmHg
   c. P 64 BPM and BP 72/50 mmHg
   d. P 58 BPM and BP 212/120 mmHg

5. A patient has fallen off a 20-foot ladder, striking his back on a railing. He is experiencing pain at the injury site and a loss of bladder control. Which part of the spinal cord is most likely affected by this mechanism?
   a. coccyx
   b. cervical
   c. sacral
   d. lumbar

6. An unrestrained driver of a small car struck a tree at high speed. He has a distended abdomen that is tender when palpated. Vital signs are pulse 120 BPM, respirations 20 breaths per minute, and blood pressure 116/90 mmHg. What would be the most likely cause of the abdominal tenderness?
   a. bacterial peritonitis
   b. abdominal muscle strain
   c. organ damage
   d. seat belt injury

7. Where would you expect to see a wound that is distal to the knee?
   a. hip
   b. stomach
   c. thigh
   d. calf

Answer questions 8–11 based on the following information.

You respond to a 63-year-old male who is complaining of a sudden onset of extreme substernal chest pain that "feels like my insides are tearing." The patient states that the pain radiates to the middle of his back between his shoulder blades.

8. From which condition is this patient most likely suffering?
   a. dissecting aortic aneurysm
   b. abdominal aortic aneurysm
   c. acute arterial occlusion
   d. acute pulmonary embolism

9. Which of the following is a predisposing factor for this patient's condition?
   a. hypotension
   b. hypertension
   c. angina pectoris
   d. myocardial infarction

10. Which of the following medications may be ordered by medical control to treat this patient?
   a. dopamine
   b. atropine sulfate
   c. morphine sulfate
   d. isoproterenol

11. Progression of this condition may cause which of the following?
   a. stroke, pericardial tamponade, acute myocardial infarction
   b. acute arterial occlusion, acute pulmonary embolism, encephalitis
   c. deep venous thrombosis, varicose veins, arterial atherosclerotic disease
   d. arterial atherosclerotic disease, pulmonary embolism, acute arterial occlusion

12. Your patient has survived a vehicle rollover in which another passenger in the vehicle died. He is alert and not complaining of pain. His vital signs are pulse 100 BPM, systolic BP 90 mmHg, and respirations 28 breaths per minute. After taking vital signs, which of the following is the correct order of procedures?
   a. Complete a detailed physical exam, stabilize his injuries, and transport.
   b. Quickly immobilize him using the long backboard as a splint and transport.
   c. Perform a focused physical exam, splint all extremity fractures, and transport.
   d. Immobilize, complete a focused physical exam of any injuries, and then transport.

13. Which statement about motorcycle crashes is correct?
   a. They seldom result in severe trauma, unless the motorcycle is operated at high speeds.
   b. Helmet use can reduce the incidence and severity of head injury.
   c. Helmet use can reduce the incidence and severity of spinal injury.
   d. Leather clothing cannot protect the rider against soft-tissue injury.

14. Which of the following is indicated by a positive Battle's sign?
   a. basilar skull fracture
   b. orbital skull fracture
   c. subarachnoid hemorrhage
   d. cervical spinal trauma

15. Your patient is a car-crash victim who was unconscious prior to your arrival, but is now awake. As you examine the patient, you notice that he is becoming disoriented. Which of the following conditions should you suspect?
   a. basilar skull fracture
   b. epidural hematoma formation
   c. concussion with awakening
   d. inner-ear injury

16. In response to pain, your trauma patient opens her eyes, withdraws her hand, and speaks only in garbled sounds. What is her Glasgow Coma Scale score?
   a. 5
   b. 7
   c. 8
   d. 11

17. Your trauma patient is agitated and apprehensive. She is increasingly cyanotic, and breath sounds are rapidly diminishing over her left lung. She is exhibiting signs and symptoms of shock. You should suspect which of the following?
   a. hemothorax
   b. tension pneumothorax
   c. cardiac tamponade
   d. flail chest

18. A child has third-degree burns over the front of her trunk and the entire front of her right arm. According to the rule of nines, the burns affect what percentage of her body surface area?
   a. 18.5%
   b. 22.5%
   c. 25%
   d. 27%

19. Your patient is a 34-year-old woman who has been in an automobile crash. Her vital signs are respiratory rate 34 with normal chest wall expansion, systolic blood pressure 78, capillary refill delayed, and a Glasgow Coma Scale score of 10. This patient's Revised Trauma Score is which of the following?
   a. 5
   b. 6
   c. 9
   d. 10

20. Which group of vital sign changes is associated with Cushing's reflex?
   a. decreased blood pressure, decreased pulse rate, decreased respiratory rate, decreased temperature
   b. increased blood pressure, decreased pulse rate, decreased respiratory rate, increased temperature
   c. decreased blood pressure, increased pulse rate, increased respiratory rate, decreased temperature
   d. increased blood pressure, increased pulse rate, increased respiratory rate, increased temperature

21. When caring for a patient with a pulmonary contusion, it is essential not to perform which of the following?
   a. Place the patient in a supine position.
   b. Overinflate the patient's lungs.
   c. Overload the patient with IV fluids.
   d. Perform an endotracheal intubation.

22. You suspect that a trauma patient has a pelvic injury. She is cool and diaphoretic. Her heart rate is 134 BPM and her blood pressure is 74/48 mmHg. Which of the following procedures is most appropriate in the management of her condition?
   a. Run one large-bore IV wide open and inflate the legs on the PASG.
   b. Run two large-bore IVs wide open and consider application of the PASG.
   c. Transport in a position of comfort.
   d. Perform the detailed assessment prior to transport.

23. A patient has been stabbed in the back. Which of the following signs would most likely make you suspect that the patient has a kidney injury?
- **a.** abdominal tenderness
- **b.** hematuria
- **c.** thirst
- **d.** ecchymosis of the flank

24. Your patient is a 24-year-old female who shows signs and symptoms of pelvic inflammatory disease. What is the goal of prehospital care for this patient?
- **a.** Begin definitive therapy on the scene prior to initiating your transport.
- **b.** Perform a complete physical exam to identify associated medical problems.
- **c.** Make the patient as comfortable as possible and transport to the hospital.
- **d.** Begin the identification of all the patient's previous sexual contacts.

25. Which of the following factors would normally cause a decrease in a patient's respiratory rate?
- **a.** aspirin overdose
- **b.** sleep
- **c.** fever
- **d.** hypoxia

26. While ventilating a patient with a bag valve mask, you note decreasing compliance. How should you react to this finding?
- **a.** Stop using the bag valve mask and intubate the patient.
- **b.** Request permission to sedate the patient with morphine.
- **c.** Assess the cause of this finding and try to correct it.
- **d.** Continue ventilation with BVM and increase the tidal volume; this is a normal finding.

27. What would a pulse oximetry reading of 88% indicate for your patient with acute respiratory distress?
- **a.** normal oxygenation
- **b.** mild hypoxia
- **c.** moderate hypoxia
- **d.** severe hypoxia

28. The primary use of Magill forceps in the field is to
- **a.** directly remove a visible foreign-body obstruction.
- **b.** open the airway of a patient with suspected neck trauma.
- **c.** move the tongue aside during attempts at intubation.
- **d.** aid in removal of an esophageal obturator airway in the field.

29. Which of the following signs most likely indicates imminent birth?
- **a.** painful uterine contractions
- **b.** urge to have a bowel movement
- **c.** ruptured membranes
- **d.** dilation of the cervix

30. Which of the following is a sign of esophageal intubation?
- **a.** air leak heard over the trachea
- **b.** breath sounds absent on the left
- **c.** bilateral chest wall expansion
- **d.** abdominal movement with ventilation

Answer questions 31 and 32 based on the following information.

You are called to the home of a 68-year-old female who is complaining of severe dyspnea. She states that it started about 45 minutes ago and has been getting progressively worse. She has a cardiac history but denies chest pain at this time. Her breathing is very congested. During your assessment, you notice accessory muscle use and bilateral crackles.

31. From which of the following conditions is this patient most likely suffering?
   a. pulmonary embolism
   b. acute pulmonary edema
   c. pneumonia
   d. lung cancer

32. In addition to oxygen, this patient should also be treated with which of the following medications?
   a. albuterol
   b. dopamine
   c. lidocaine
   d. morphine sulfate

33. A pregnant patient complains of painful, irregular labor contractions. The patient states that she is 37 weeks pregnant and her amniotic membranes ruptured two days ago. Based on this information, you would perform which of the following?
   a. Perform a field delivery.
   b. Initiate immediate transport.
   c. Inform the patient that she is experiencing Braxton-Hicks contractions.
   d. Tell the patient to call when her contractions become regular.

34. Which drug is an example of a beta2-agonist?
   a. aminophylline
   b. ipratropium
   c. labetalol
   d. albuterol

35. What is the condition that is present when the pleural space expands because air enters from an interior wound?
   a. closed pneumothorax
   b. open pneumothorax
   c. tension pneumothorax
   d. traumatic asphyxia

36. To which of the following does the term *stridor* refer?
   a. a rattling sound associated with fluid in the upper airway
   b. a whistling sound heard upon expiration in asthma patients
   c. a gurgling sound resulting from fluid in the lower airways
   d. a high-pitched sound upon inspiration from airway obstruction

37. A patient who is 37 weeks pregnant is having contractions and states that her water broke about 20 minutes ago. The vaginal exam reveals that the baby's foot is present in the birth canal. Your next action would be to
   a. move the patient to the cot and initiate rapid transport.
   b. turn the mother onto her stomach and prepare for a field delivery.
   c. apply downward pressure on the symphysis pubis to delay delivery.
   d. place the mother on her left side and prepare for a field delivery.

38. What is the primary treatment for a patient with chronic emphysema who is NOT severely hypoxic?
   a. ventilation with high-flow oxygen via mask
   b. administration of low-flow oxygen via cannula
   c. nasotracheal intubation and high-flow oxygen
   d. orotracheal intubation and high-flow oxygen

39. Epinephrine 1:1,000 may be indicated for which of the following conditions?
   a. asthma
   b. epiglottitis
   c. pertussis
   d. emphysema

40. You are on the scene of a vehicle crash involving a bus. As triage officer, the first patient you encounter is sitting on the ground, conscious, confused, and breathing 40 times per minute. She states that she was thrown out of her seat and struck the side of her head. Your next action would be to
   a. apply oxygen by nonrebreather mask.
   b. check the radial pulse rate.
   c. classify the patient as *immediate* (red).
   d. apply a *hold* (green) triage tag.

Answer questions 41–43 based on the following information.

You are called to the home of a 17-year-old female who was found by her parents hanging from a rope in the garage. Her father cut down the patient approximately six minutes prior to your arrival; however, the patient is unconscious and unresponsive to pain or voice. She is breathing spontaneously, but has coarse inspiratory stridor.

41. What is the most probable cause of the inspiratory stridor?
   a. a trachea that is crushed or torn
   b. a cervical spine lesion from trauma
   c. bronchoconstriction due to trauma
   d. a foreign-body airway obstruction

42. Upon examination of the patient's upper chest and neck, you note the presence of a large swollen area that extends from her throat to her shoulder. When you press on this area, you feel crackles under the skin. What is this condition called?
   a. traumatic asphyxia
   b. laryngeal crepitus
   c. subcutaneous emphysema
   d. subcutaneous embolism

43. Which of the following is an appropriate treatment for this patient?
   a. crichothyrotomy or transtracheal jet insufflation
   b. airway management by the least invasive means
   c. laryngoscopy to determine the extent of damage
   d. administration of epinephrine to reverse airway swelling

44. Your partner and you are evaluating a patient experiencing a behavioral emergency. Your patient is visibly upset and is pacing back and forth. He is verbally confrontational and his hands are in fists. At times, he displays aggressive actions, both physical and verbal. Which of the following actions is most appropriate for this situation?
   a. Observe the scene for danger.
   b. Conduct a patient assessment.
   c. Obtain information from bystanders.
   d. Physically restrain the patient.

45. A critically traumatized 18-year-old male is trapped. It will be at least 15 minutes before he is freed. The community hospital is 20 minutes away by ground. A medical helicopter can be to the scene in eight minutes. A Level I Trauma Center is one hour away by ground. Given the situation, which is the best mode of transport for this patient?
   a. Transport the patient by ground to the community hospital, and then transfer the patient to the trauma center by air.
   b. Transport the patient by ground to the Level I Trauma Center.
   c. Fly the patient from the scene to the community hospital.
   d. Fly the patient from the scene to the Level I Trauma Center.

46. What is the first sign of laryngeal edema in a patient suffering from anaphylaxis?
   a. wheezing
   b. coughing
   c. hoarseness
   d. dyspnea

47. What does the disease process of emphysema cause within the lung tissues?
   a. a buildup of fluid due to increased capillary permeability
   b. deflation of a portion of the lung due to the rupture of a bleb
   c. bronchoconstriction due to increased airway resistance
   d. a loss of elasticity in the alveoli due to prolonged insult

Answer questions 48–53 based on the following information.

You are called to the home of a 78-year-old male who is having difficulty breathing. The patient is sitting upright in a tripod position. You note profound accessory muscle use. His skin is pale, cool, and clammy. Vital signs are: blood pressure 180/72, heart rate 90 BPM, and respiratory rate 40 breaths per minute. Breathing is shallow and labored with a coarse rattling sound during expiration. Auscultation reveals coarse crackles to the nipple line with no air movement in the bases.

The patient can speak only in one- or two-word sentences. Family members inform you that the patient was sleeping when this episode began and that this has happened several times since his acute myocardial infarction (AMI) one year ago. He has mild pedal edema. Neck veins are nondistended. His family first noticed the patient having dyspnea about 25–30 minutes ago.

48. This patient is exhibiting the signs and symptoms of which of the following diseases?
   a. chronic bronchitis
   b. emphysema
   c. congestive heart failure
   d. status asthmaticus

49. Which of the following medication should be used for this patient?
   a. albuterol
   b. nitrous oxide
   c. dobutamine
   d. morphine sulfate

50. A patient with the symptoms and history described may exhibit which of the following symptoms prior to an acute onset?
   a. orthostatic hypotension
   b. paroxysmal nocturnal dyspnea
   c. cough and fever
   d. headache

51. Priorities for the management of this patient include all EXCEPT which one of the following?
a. decreasing venous return to the heart
b. increasing venous return to the heart
c. decreasing myocardial oxygen demand
d. improving oxygenation and ventilation

52. This patient would most likely benefit from which of the following?
a. moving him to a supine position
b. assisting him in walking to the ambulance
c. having him breathe deeply into a paper bag
d. giving him intermittent positive pressure ventilation

53. If this patient were experiencing right-sided heart failure, you would expect to find all EXCEPT which one of the following?
a. tachycardia
b. profound peripheral edema
c. jugular venous distention
d. syncope

54. Which of the following best describes an isotonic solution?
a. It has an electrolyte composition like that of blood plasma.
b. It is used only in patients who are severely dehydrated.
c. It has a higher solute composition than the body cells.
d. It has a lower solute composition than the body cells.

55. A patient has been violently beaten. Which of the following statements is true surrounding EMS-provided care?
a. Evidence preservation should be the first priority.
b. Latex gloves will prevent you from smudging fingerprints.
c. Statements made by the patient should be recorded in the report.
d. Bloody clothing should be placed in plastic bags.

56. An injury to the ligaments surrounding a joint that is marked by pain, swelling, and bruising is called which of the following?
a. sprain
b. strain
c. dislocation
d. arthritis

57. Why is morphine sulfate used in the management of AMI patients?
a. It helps distinguish between angina pectoris and AMI.
b. It relieves pain and reduces myocardial oxygen demand.
c. It decreases the likelihood of ventricular dysrhythmias.
d. It is an alternative therapy for patients allergic to lidocaine.

58. Paroxysmal nocturnal dyspnea (PND) is commonly a sign of which of the following conditions?
a. myocardial infarction
b. ruptured aortic aneurysm
c. left-sided heart failure
d. right-sided heart failure

59. You are inserting a nasotracheal tube when you begin to hear the sound of the patient's breathing. Your next action would be to perform which of the following?
   a. Inflate the distal cuff and secure the tube.
   b. Wait until the patient inhales to insert the tube farther.
   c. Pull back on the tube and secure with tape.
   d. Attach an end-tidal CO_2 detector to confirm placement.

60. What is the initial electrical treatment for a patient with third-degree AV block who is symptomatic?
   a. insertion of a demand pacemaker
   b. unsynchronized cardioversion
   c. transcutaneous cardiac pacing
   d. synchronized cardioversion

61. A patient suspected of having an abdominal aortic aneurysm will receive oxygen, an IV, ECG monitoring, and rapid transport as part of his or her treatment. What else should you do when treating such a patient?
   a. Consider permissive reduction of the patient's heart rate and blood pressure.
   b. Carefully palpate the abdomen.
   c. Administer dopamine or dobutamine.
   d. Administer SL nifedipine.

62. A 52-year-old male has been ejected from a car. He is apneic and has a slow pulse that was palpated at the femoral artery. Which of the following procedures would be the best way to ventilate this patient?
   a. Nasotracheally intubate the patient.
   b. Ventilate with the bag-valve mask and attach to high-flow oxygen.
   c. Apply a nonrebreather mask with high-flow oxygen.
   d. Perform immediate orotracheal intubation.

63. Vagal maneuvers are used to treat which type of dysrhythmias?
   a. premature atrial contractions
   b. ventricular tachycardia
   c. atrial fibrillation or flutter
   d. paroxysmal supraventricular tachycardia

64. What is the length of the normal P-R interval?
   a. 0.04–0.12 seconds
   b. 0.12–0.20 seconds
   c. 0.20–0.28 seconds
   d. 0.28–0.36 seconds

65. A 3-year-old female is unresponsive and not breathing. Parents state that she was eating grapes when she suddenly made a high-pitched whistling noise and turned blue. Your immediate action would be to
   a. provide back blows and chest thrusts.
   b. start cardiopulmonary resuscitation.
   c. perform endotracheal intubation.
   d. perform abdominal thrusts.

66. While assessing a patient complaining of difficulty breathing, you note an altered mental status, stridor, chest tightness, and tachycardia. Based on these symptoms, you should suspect which of the following conditions?
   a. cerebrovascular accident (CVA)
   b. emphysema
   c. asthma attack
   d. anaphylaxis

67. Which of the following best describes the Quantron Resonance System (QRS) complex in a patient with ventricular tachycardia?
   a. absent during the cardiac cycle
   b. 0.04 and 0.12 seconds in duration
   c. greater than 0.12 seconds and uncharacteristic in shape
   d. shorter than 0.04 seconds and flattened

68. A patient with nonperfusing ventricular tachycardia would receive the same treatment as a patient with which other rhythm?
a. ventricular fibrillation
b. perfusing ventricular tachycardia
c. atrial tachycardia
d. asystole

69. Which of the following are signs and symptoms of right-side heart failure?
a. tachycardia, peripheral edema, and jugular vein distention
b. bradycardia, carotid bruits, and falling blood pressure
c. respiratory distress, hypoxia, and cyanosis
d. chest pain, pulmonary edema, and anxiety

70. A 65-year-old female is complaining of chest pressure, difficulty breathing, and is pale. She presents supine in bed. What should you do before sitting her up?
a. Check her blood pressure to make sure it is adequate.
b. Do nothing; sit her up right away.
c. Help the patient administer her own nitroglycerin tablets.
d. Check her pupils to make sure they are reactive.

71. Why are easing anxiety and relieving pain considered major goals for prehospital care of myocardial infarction (MI) patients?
a. The onset of either may signal the development of a lethal dysrhythmia.
b. Anxiety and pain often mask underlying symptoms of cardiogenic shock.
c. They may prevent the patient from cooperating with additional treatments.
d. Both anxiety and pain increase heart rate and myocardial oxygen demand.

72. Which of the following best describes a use of dopamine?
a. to decrease oxygen demand
b. to increase cardiac output
c. to reduce blood pressure
d. to prevent dysrhythmias

73. A patient is short of breath after impact with the steering wheel in a motor vehicle crash. Breath sounds are diminished on the left. Which of the following conditions is most likely the cause of the patient's complaint?
a. simple pneumothorax
b. tension pneumothorax
c. pulmonary contusion
d. cardiac tamponade

74. Some treatments for suspected MI patients mask the elevated cardiac enzyme levels that are used to diagnose MI in the hospital setting. To prevent this, you should not administer which of the following?
a. transcutaneous pacing
b. any drugs via the intramuscular (IM) route
c. any nebulized beta-agonists
d. diazepam or morphine sulfate IV

75. Your patient is a 67-year-old male who is complaining of chest pain. The chest pain continues after two doses of nitroglycerin. He reports a history of angina and says that all his previous attacks have been relieved by nitroglycerin. How should you treat this patient?
a. Take a detailed history to determine why this episode is different.
b. Treat the patient as though he is having an AMI and transport rapidly.
c. Look for signs and symptoms of decreased perfusion or cardiogenic shock.
d. Assume that his medication has expired and give two more doses from your supply.

76. What regulates the hypoxic drive?
a. low PaO_2
b. high PaO_2
c. high oxygen saturation percentage
d. low oxygen saturation percentage

77. In addition to oxygen, what is the first-line pharmacologic agent used for the treatment of malignant PVCs?
a. lidocaine
b. bretylium
c. procainamide
d. magnesium sulfate

78. Your patient, who has had a recent tracheostomy, tried to remove himself from the ventilator and dislodged the trach cannula. Subcutaneous emphysema is now evident. What should you do next?
a. Remove the tracheostomy tube and attempt to reinsert it.
b. Remove the tracheostomy tube and insert an endotracheal tube.
c. Deflate the tracheostomy cuff and ventilate around it with a BVM.
d. Continue to ventilate the patient through the tracheostomy tube.

Answer questions 79–81 based on the following information.

You are called by the police department to a neighborhood where you encounter an approximately 20- to 30-year-old male patient. The police officer states that neighbors called because the patient was "freaking out." Witnesses say they saw him smoking something just before he started acting in a bizarre manner. During your assessment, you notice that the patient is hyperactive and anxious. His pupils are dilated, and he is hypertensive and tachycardic.

79. This patient is most likely experiencing which of the following?
a. insulin shock
b. cocaine inhalation
c. narcotic inhalation
d. delirium tremens

80. The appropriate treatment for this patient consists of oxygen, IV, ECG monitoring, and which of the following?
a. transport
b. naloxone
c. activated charcoal
d. syrup of ipecac

81. When treating this patient, you should be prepared for which of the following complications?
a. tachycardia and septic shock
b. CNS depression and hypoglycemia
c. dysrhythmias and seizures
d. bradycardia and tachypnea

82. Your patient is in respiratory distress. He is exhibiting jugular venous distension. Crackles are auscultated throughout his lung fields. He is tachycardic, hypertensive, and tachypneic. Which of the following sets of treatment is indicated for this patient's presentation?
a. oxygen, morphine sulfate IM, intravenous line at 30 mL/hour, and 40 mg furosemide IV
b. oxygen, intravenous line at 30 mL/hour, nitroglycerin SL, and 40 mg furosemide IV
c. oxygen, saline lock, and 2 mg morphine sulfate IV
d. oxygen, sublingual nitroglycerin, and 40 mg furosemide IM

83. A patient is complaining of chest pressure and shortness of breath. He has jugular venous distension and pedal edema. His lung sounds are clear and equal. Which of the following conditions most likely causes these findings?
a. left-sided heart failure
b. right-sided heart failure
c. pulmonary embolus
d. cardiac asthma

84. Your patient has a suspected hand injury. How can you best immobilize the hand in the position of function?
a. Tape it flat against the chest with the fingers extended outward together.
b. Put the arm into a sling and swathe and allow the hand to dangle naturally.
c. Place a roll of gauze bandage into the palm and secure the hand to a splint.
d. Secure the hand to a padded splint with the hand clenched into a fist.

85. You are caring for a patient whose finger was just cut off in an accident. What should you do with the amputated finger?
a. Place the severed finger in a plastic bag and immerse the bag in cold water.
b. Immerse the severed finger directly into a pail of ice-cold normal saline solution.
c. Bandage the severed finger in sterile gauze and place it in a plastic bag with ice.
d. Bandage the hand with the severed finger placed back into its normal position.

86. Which of the following is NOT characteristic of a mild or moderate pit viper envenomation?
a. bruising located around the wound site
b. systemic effects like nausea or vomiting
c. localized edema at the wound site
d. little or no pain felt by the patient

87. How should you treat a patient who has sustained dry lime burns to the hand and arm?
a. Use a neutralizing acid to offset the effect of the chemical burn.
b. Brush the lime away and then flood the skin with cool water.
c. Immediately immerse the injured limb in a bucket of cold water.
d. Use alcohol to dissolve the lime and then flood with cool water.

88. Diabetic patients may develop hypoglycemia if they take too much insulin or if they
a. exercise too much with limited food intake.
b. overeat and do not exercise enough.
c. sit in a chair for prolonged periods of time.
d. inject their insulin directly into a vein.

89. With which of the following conditions is central neurogenic hyperventilation commonly associated?
a. diabetes mellitus
b. CNS trauma
c. pulmonary edema
d. COPD

90. A patient is in respiratory distress. She has a valid DNR order. Which of the following treatments is correct?
a. Nothing should be done to the patient in this situation.
b. Provide oxygen and a nebulized albuterol treatment.
c. Administer 2 L of oxygen via a nasal cannula.
d. Initiate a direct laryngoscopy and intubation.

91. You have secured the airway and immobilized the cervical spine for your patient with an altered mental status. What is your next priority of care?
 a. Draw blood for glucose assessment and establish an IV.
 b. Assess deformities, contusions, abrasions, punctures/penetrations, burns, tenderness, lacerations, and swelling (DCAP-BTLS), looking for any hidden injuries.
 c. Administer naloxone via the IV and IM glucagon.
 d. Hyperventilate with O_2 and administer dexamethasone.

92. You are called to the home of a 36-year-old man who is having a seizure. His wife reports that he has not taken his "seizure pills" lately and has had three seizures in a row without regaining consciousness. You have secured the airway and are now ventilating with the bag-valve mask. What should you do next?
 a. Draw blood, administer dextrose, and transport immediately.
 b. Monitor blood glucose level and administer naloxone and thiamine.
 c. Secure the patient to a long spine board until the seizures are over.
 d. Begin an IV, monitor cardiac rhythm, and administer diazepam.

93. What is the primary treatment for severe anaphylaxis in an adult?
 a. 0.3–0.5 mg of epinephrine 1:10,000 given intravenously
 b. 0.1–0.3 mg of epinephrine 1:10,000 given subcutaneously
 c. 0.3–0.5 mg of epinephrine 1:1,000 given intravenously
 d. 0.1–0.3 mg of epinephrine 1:1,000 given subcutaneously

94. Which of the following patients is considered to be at high risk for a heat-related emergency?
 a. 29-year-old amputee
 b. 48-year-old police officer
 c. 17-year-old athlete
 d. 78-year-old diabetic

95. Which of the following is a late sign of hypoxia in children?
 a. tachypnea
 b. hypotension
 c. tachycardia
 d. bradycardia

96. What is the most important treatment consideration for a patient who is suffering from decompression sickness?
 a. Have suction equipment ready because vomiting is common.
 b. Monitor the ECG and be prepared to defibrillate as necessary.
 c. Provide high-concentration oxygen with a nonrebreather mask.
 d. Administer nitrous oxide or morphine sulfate as needed to control pain.

97. When interviewing patients who are distraught or potentially violent, you should do all EXCEPT which one of the following?
 a. Remove the patient from the crisis situation as quickly as possible.
 b. Encourage the patient to explain the situation in his or her own words.
 c. Firmly tell the patient whenever he or she is distorting reality.
 d. Avoid arguing with or shouting at the person who is distraught.

98. Lifting improperly may most likely result in an injury to which region of the back?
   a. cervical
   b. thoracic
   c. lumbar
   d. sacral

99. After experiencing a sudden syncopal episode, a 41-year-old female is complaining of pleuritic chest pain and shortness of breath. Her vital signs are RR 28 breaths per minute, P 126 BPM, and BP 88/60 mmHg. The pulse oximeter reads 89% on high-flow oxygen. Her breath sounds are clear. Which of the following conditions best describes the patient's signs and symptoms?
   a. pulmonary embolism
   b. pulmonary edema
   c. chronic bronchitis
   d. acute asthma

100. What is the management for a patient with a head injury and an unusual respiratory pattern?
   a. positioning in the left lateral recumbent position
   b. administration of oxygen and methylprednisolone
   c. rapid transport because of possible brain stem injury
   d. intubation and hyperventilation to reduce ICP

Answer questions 101 and 102 based on the following information.

You respond to a 56-year-old male who appears to be intoxicated. He is belligerent and disoriented. He has a laceration on his forehead. You have made several attempts to convince him of the need for treatment, but he refuses treatment or transport.

101. Given this situation, you should perform which of the following?
   a. Let him sign a refusal form and return to service.
   b. Call medical direction for advice and guidance.
   c. Transport the patient against his will in restraints.
   d. Bandage the laceration and then leave the scene.

102. Regardless of any of the options considered in the previous question, the patient continues to insist he does not need medical attention. In this situation, which of the following is most important?
   a. Obtain a signed refusal form and return to service as soon as possible.
   b. Continue to insist that the patient accompany you to the hospital for care.
   c. Properly document your advice to the patient and request law enforcement to respond.
   d. Restrain the patient in the supine position and transport him immediately.

103. You are called to treat a patient who is unconscious and only responsive to painful stimuli. Which of the following treatment modalities is appropriate for this patient?
   a. 25 gm of 50% dextrose slow IV push, 2 mg naloxone IV, and transport to a detoxification center
   b. blood glucose test, dextrose (if indicated), thiamine, monitoring, oxygen, IV, and rapid transport
   c. oxygen, IV fluid bolus titrated to a systolic BP of 100–110 mmHg, naloxone, and rapid transport
   d. 1,000 mL lactated Ringer's IV solution, oxygen, ECG monitoring, and transport to an emergency department

104. During a basketball game, an 18-year-old male is complaining of sudden shortness of breath and sharp chest pain that increases with inspiration. He is alert, warm, and diaphoretic. His vital signs are RR 24 breaths per minute, P 100 BPM, and BP 122/84 mmHg. His breath sounds are diminished in the lower right lung field. He denies any medical history, does not smoke, and takes no medication. Which of the following conditions best describes the patient's signs and symptoms?

a. pulmonary embolism
b. simple pneumothorax
c. asthma
d. COPD

105. A 64-year-old male complains of weakness and dizziness. He is anxious, with a patent airway and adequate breathing. His pulse is rapid. His skin is cool and diaphoretic. Auscultation of the lung fields or lungs reveals bilateral crackles. His vital signs are pulse 156 BPM, respiration 28 breaths per minute, blood pressure 82/60 mmHg, and SpO_2 92%. His ECG is depicted in Figure 4.1. What is the best treatment for this patient?

a. to decrease the atrial rate
b. to restore a normal sinus rhythm
c. to decrease the ventricular rate
d. to increase cardiac contractility

106. Which of the following statements regarding a spontaneous pneumothorax is true?

a. It usually requires prehospital chest decompression.
b. It is usually limited to only 20% of the lung and is well tolerated by the patient.
c. It often progresses to a tension pneumothorax if not relieved.
d. It usually occurs in individuals more than 50 years of age who are otherwise healthy.

107. Where is the best place to assess for cyanosis in an infant or child?

a. oral mucosa
b. nail beds
c. soles of the feet
d. area around the eyes

108. What volume of fluid bolus should be given initially to a severely dehydrated child?

a. 20 mL/kg
b. 30 mL/kg
c. 40 mL/kg
d. 50 mL/kg

Figure 4.1

Answer questions 109–112 based on the following information.

> You are called to the home of a 21-year-old female in active labor. She is two weeks from her expected due date and is having contractions of 1.5 minutes duration that are three minutes apart. This is her second pregnancy. Her first child was delivered vaginally at full term.

109. What is your first course of action for this patient?
- **a.** Place her on the stretcher in high Fowler's or comfortable position and examine her for crowning.
- **b.** Place her in the left-lateral recumbent position, apply oxygen, and transport her immediately.
- **c.** Call her obstetrician and advise him or her that the birth is imminent.
- **d.** Place her in position of comfort with a sanitary napkin over her vagina and transport rapidly.

110. Your patient suddenly tells you she feels something slippery between her legs. Upon visual examination, you notice a two-inch segment of the umbilical cord protruding from the vagina. What is this condition called?
- **a.** prolapsed cord
- **b.** abruptio umbilicus
- **c.** placenta previa
- **d.** abruptio previa

111. Which of the following is NOT an appropriate treatment option for this patient?
- **a.** providing high-flow oxygen and rapidly transporting the mother in the knee-chest position
- **b.** taking pressure off the cord by placing your fingers into the vagina and gently lifting the infant
- **c.** wrapping the cord in a moist sterile dressing, providing supplemental oxygen, and transporting quickly
- **d.** placing the mother in the right-lateral recumbent position, and transporting immediately

112. You are ready to transport this patient. If the umbilical cord is still exposed, how can you use it to evaluate the infant's perfusion?
- **a.** Gently feel the cord for pulsations to determine the infant's heart rate.
- **b.** Determine the infant's temperature by feeling the cord for changes.
- **c.** Look at the umbilical cord for color changes, with blue indicating hypoxia.
- **d.** Attach a pulse oximetry lead to the cord and determine the oxygen saturation.

113. You arrive at the scene of an imminent delivery in the field. The first responder, who called for assistance, reports that the patient is a 32-year-old female who is "G4 P3." What does this mean?
- **a.** The patient is pregnant for the seventh time and has three living children.
- **b.** The patient's cervix has dilated a total of four centimeters in three hours.
- **c.** The patient has been pregnant four times and delivered three live infants.
- **d.** The patient has had four rounds of contractions timed three minutes apart.

114. What does the term *effacement* refer to?
   a. direction the fetus is facing during the birth
   b. position of the fetus in the uterus prior to birth
   c. thinning of the cervix during the first stage of labor
   d. opening of the cervix during the last stage of labor

115. Your patient is a 33-year-old woman who is nine months pregnant. She complains of severe abdominal pain and abdominal tenderness. She reports there is no vaginal bleeding at this time. What should you suspect?
   a. abruptio placentae
   b. placenta previa
   c. threatened abortion
   d. preeclampsia

116. Which of the following signs and symptoms would be present in a pregnant patient with preeclampsia?
   a. high blood pressure, normal pulse rate, and normal respiratory rate
   b. high blood pressure, headaches, edema, and visual disturbances
   c. high blood pressure, edema, excessive weight gain, and seizures
   d. high blood pressure, abdominal pain, and bright-red bleeding

117. When does the third stage of labor begin?
   a. when contractions are five minutes apart
   b. when the cervix is fully dilated
   c. immediately upon the birth of the baby
   d. as the placenta is delivered

118. What is the correct procedure for cutting the umbilical cord after the birth of the baby?
   a. Milk the cord of all blood and cut it no more than 5 cm from the infant.
   b. Clamp the cord close to the infant and cut it between the infant and the clamp.
   c. Clamp the cord in two places and cut it near the infant and near the placenta.
   d. Clamp the cord in two places 5 cm apart and cut it between the clamps.

119. What is the appropriate range for the heart rate of a healthy neonate immediately after birth?
   a. 80–100 beats per minute
   b. 100–120 beats per minute
   c. 120–150 beats per minute
   d. 150–180 beats per minute

120. You would perform chest compressions on any newborn whose heart rate is less than how many beats per minute?
   a. 120
   b. 100
   c. 80
   d. 60

121. Medications and drugs are most often delivered to a newborn through the use of which circulatory vessel?
   a. umbilical artery
   b. umbilical vein
   c. ductus arteriosus
   d. jugular vein

Answer questions 122–124 based on the following information.

You respond to a 2-year-old female who is post-ictal following seizure activity. The patient's parents report that the child was sleeping when she began to shake and turn blue. She has had a runny nose, but she has had no medications lately. There is no history of seizures.

122. This patient is most likely suffering from which condition?
  a. juvenile diabetes
  b. a hypoglycemic seizure
  c. an anaphylactic seizure
  d. a febrile seizure

123. Which of the following vital signs would you expect this patient to have?
  a. increased body temperature, tachycardia, and tachypnea
  b. normal temperature, normal blood pressure, and bradycardia
  c. increased temperature, increased blood pressure, and bradycardia
  d. normal body temperature, tachycardia, and bradypnea

124. What would be the appropriate treatment if this patient continues in a prolonged postictal state?
  a. obtain blood glucose readings and administer 25% dextrose as needed
  b. apply ice packs to the armpits and groin
  c. remove the child's excess clothing, administer oxygen and an IV, and transport
  d. administer high-concentration oxygen, diazepam, and naloxone, and transport

125. You are caring for a 63-year-old male patient with renal failure. He is pulseless and apneic. Figure 4.2 depicts his ECG. Appropriate treatment for this patient would include all EXCEPT which one of the following?
  a. immediate defibrillation
  b. administration of dextrose and sodium bicarbonate
  c. administration of lidocaine or amiodarone
  d. administration of sodium bicarbonate and calcium gluconate

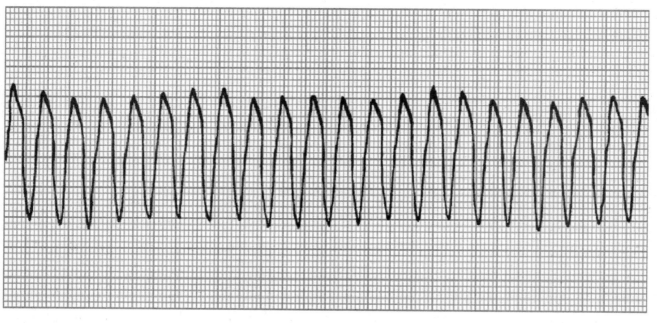

Figure 4.2

126. A patient with a past medical history (PMH) of emphysema experiences a sudden onset of respiratory distress and sharp chest pain. His skin is warm and dry. His breath sounds are diminished on the left side. Your strongest suspicion is which of the following conditions?
a. pulmonary embolism
b. pneumonia
c. pneumothorax
d. chronic bronchitis

127. What feature does a type II ambulance exhibit?
a. conventional cab-and-chassis truck
b. standard van, usually with a raised roof
c. special cab-forward van with an integral body
d. modified suburban vehicle that can provide transport

128. Which legal document does not specify what type of treatment a patient does and does not want to receive?
a. a do-not-resuscitate (DNR) order
b. a living will
c. an advance directive
d. a durable power of attorney

129. In most states, at what age is a person considered capable of giving consent to treatment?
a. 15
b. 16
c. 18
d. 21

130. An unconscious patient has snoring respirations. When should this condition be corrected?
a. simultaneously with the physical exam
b. on completion of the initial assessment
c. on assessing for the presence of a pulse
d. before evaluating the respiratory status

131. You are caring for a female patient who was struck by an automobile. She opens her eyes to voice command only, localizes pain when you pinch her arm, and is awake but confused. What is her Glasgow Coma Scale score?
a. 6
b. 8
c. 12
d. 14

132. You are the first paramedic unit to arrive on the scene of a multi-injury bus crash. What is your first responsibility?
a. assume command of the incident and give a preliminary report to dispatch
b. wait until an incident commander arrives on scene and then follow his or her direction
c. extract patients from the bus and triage them into categories by color or priority
d. review and evaluate the efficiency of site operations up until your arrival

133. A patient presents with shallow breaths at a rate of six per minute. What should you do next?
a. Initiate IV therapy.
b. Check for carotid and radial pulses.
c. Administer positive-pressure ventilation with a BVM.
d. Identify the specific cause of the respiratory distress.

134. Under the START method, which patient would be categorized as immediate without further assessment?
a. male with no respiratory effort
b. female with a respiratory rate of 12/min.
c. male with a respiratory rate of 28/min.
d. female with a respiratory rate of 38/min.

135. What is the difference between bulimia and anorexia nervosa?
  a. They are basically the same disorder.
  b. Bulimia is an intense fear of obesity, whereas anorexia is the insatiable craving for food.
  c. Anorexia is less severe and rarely life threatening.
  d. Bulimia is more often associated with binge eating.

136. Which patient is likely to need rapid transport to a trauma center rather than assessment and stabilization on the scene?
  a. male, age 56, ejected from a crashed vehicle with a flail chest
  b. female, age 60, first degree burns to 10% BSA on her chest and abdomen
  c. male, age 28, fell 10 feet from a platform onto a pile of mulch
  d. female, age 46, struck by car traveling 10 mph, no penetrating injuries

137. For which procedure is it necessary to wear a mask and protective eyewear?
  a. endotracheal intubation
  b. starting a peripheral IV
  c. giving an IM or SC injection
  d. cleaning a contaminated ambulance

138. What is the most common job-related source of HIV infections among healthcare workers?
  a. assisting at emergency childbirth
  b. direct contact with a patient's skin
  c. an accidental needle stick
  d. breathing contaminated air

139. What is the leading cause of death among the elderly?
  a. metastatic cancer
  b. respiratory disease
  c. accidents and falls
  d. cardiac disease

140. Your patient is 2 years old. How can you reassure her before listening to her chest with your stethoscope?
  a. Explain in detail exactly how the stethoscope works.
  b. Gain her trust by letting her listen to your chest first.
  c. Hold up the stethoscope so she can see that it will not hurt her.
  d. Let her take the stethoscope apart so she is not afraid.

141. Battle's sign and periorbital ecchymosis are classic signs of which of the following conditions?
  a. a basilar skull fracture
  b. intracerebral hemorrhage
  c. a subdural hematoma
  d. a depressed skull fracture

142. There are many factors to consider when assessing a patient for suicide risk. Which of the following accurately accounts for one suicide risk factor?
  a. Young women commit suicide more often than young men do.
  b. Generally, men attempt suicide more often than women do.
  c. People with a previous history of suicide attempts are more likely to commit suicide.
  d. Suicide is the leading cause of death in Hispanic women under 30.

143. Which transmission system would you need to be able to carry on a two-way conversation with a physician while also transmitting telemetry?
  a. simplex
  b. duplex
  c. multiplex
  d. quadriplex

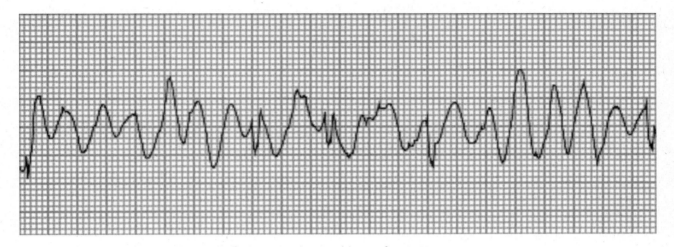

Figure 4.3 Reprinted by permission from Mauvila.com (2004, fig. 9-2).

144. What is the rhythm in Figure 4.3?
   a. PVC couplets
   b. ventricular fibrillation
   c. ventricular tachycardia
   d. supraventricular tachycardia

145. What is the location of the infarct in the 12-lead ECG in Figure 4.4?
   a. inferior wall MI
   b. septal wall MI
   c. left bundle branch block
   d. lateral wall MI

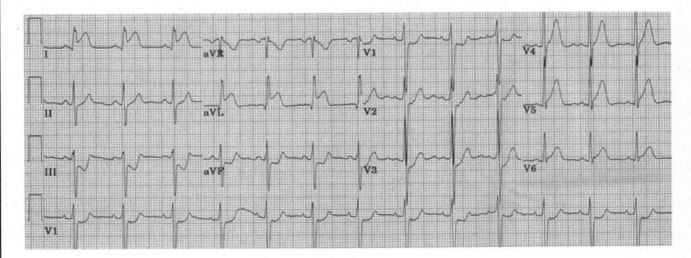

Figure 4.4 Reprinted by permission from Ed Burns (Example 1).

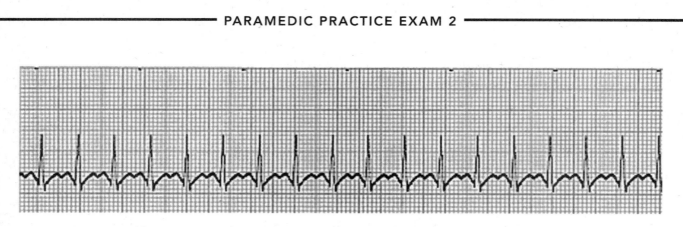

Figure 4.5 Reprinted by permission from Ambulance Technician Study (2012).

146. You are treating a 52-year-old male patient who is complaining of excruciating chest pain and shortness of breath. The patient has a pulse of 180 BPM, blood pressure of 134/86 mmHg, and respirations of 24 breaths per minute. His skin is cool, dry, and pink. You place the patient on the monitor and obtain the ECG in Figure 4.5. What is the correct order of treatment for this patient?
   a. vagal maneuvers, 0.5 mg atropine IV, transcutaneous pacing
   b. 1.0–1.5 mg/kg lidocaine IV, defibrillation
   c. vagal maneuvers, 6 mg adenosine rapid IV, 6 mg adenosine rapid IV, 12 mg adenosine rapid IV, synchronized cardioversion
   d. vagal maneuvers, 12 mg adenosine

147. What is thedentify rhythm in Figure 4.6?
   a. sinus bradycardia
   b. second-degree AV block (Mobitz type II)
   c. sinus tachycardia
   d. third-degree AV block with junctional escape beats

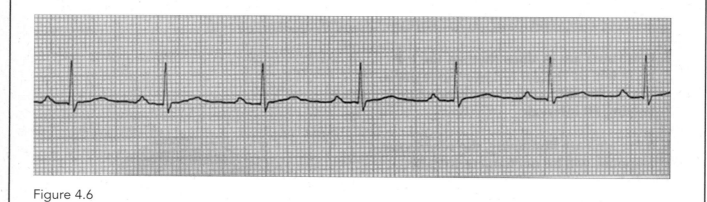

Figure 4.6

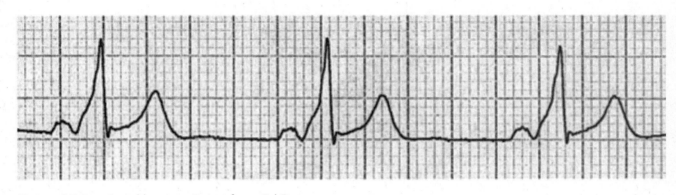

Figure 4.7 Reprinted by permission from Ed Burns.

148. What does the delta wave in the ECG in Figure 4.7 indicate?
   a. Wolff-Parkinson-White syndrome
   b. hypothermia
   c. hyperkalemia
   d. hypokalemia

149. Which of the following is a reversal agent for succinylcholine?
   a. nalaxone
   b. neostigmine
   c. sugammadex
   d. There is no reversal agent.

150. You are adjusting the positive end-expiratory pressure (PEEP) on your transport ventilator. Which of the following ranges best represents normal physiologic PEEP?
   a. 0–2 cm H_2O
   b. 3–5 cm H_2O
   c. 5–10 cm H_2O
   d. 10–20 cm H_2O

Answers

1. b. The airway is always given first priority, but in this case, since the patient is talking, the first step in his assessment and care would be to stabilize the cervical spine as you begin your ABC assessment.

2. b. Snoring indicates that the airway is partially obstructed by the patient's tongue. Clear the airway first by positioning with the jaw-thrust/chin-lift maneuver or by inserting a nasopharyngeal airway. An oropharyngeal airway is not indicated due to the patient's level of consciousness (LOC). Cervical stabilization takes place prior to beginning your ABC assessment. Head-tilt/chin-lift is not advisable due to the possibility of c-spine injury.

3. c. The START method quickly reviews three categories to determine patient priority: respirations, pulse, and mental status. After respiratory status is assessed, the basis for judging a patient's hemodynamic status is presence or absence of a radial pulse, or skin color and temperature. This patient is showing signs of shock.

4. a. By definition, compensatory shock means that in the presence of a hypoperfusion state, the body maintains its blood pressure to the brain. One way to maintain this condition is to increase the heart rate. Choice **a** satisfies both of these conditions.

5. c. Nerves that assist in bladder control exit from the sacral spine, located above the coccyx.

6. c. Organ damage from the mechanism of injury may result in inflammation and bleeding, resulting in the compensatory vital signs.

7. d. *Distal* refers to a location that is further from the trunk of the body than the reference point.

8. a. This patient is exhibiting classic signs and symptoms for a dissecting aortic aneurysm. The tearing sensation occurs when the intimal linings of the aorta are separated as blood collects between the tissues.

9. b. Hypertension is present in 75–85% of dissecting aortic aneurysm cases.

10. c. Morphine sulfate is the appropriate medication for this patient. Medications that increase cardiac rate, output, function, or contractile force are contraindicated while the dissection is occurring.

11. a. The conditions in choice **a** are all consequences of further dissection. Other conditions also include syncope, heart failure, absent or reduced pulses, and death.

12. b. Even though the patient's condition appears to be stable, the mechanism of injury indicates that serious underlying injuries, such as internal bleeding, may be present. Immobilize him quickly using the long board as a full-body splint. Transport immediately in this case. You can perform additional assessments or treatments while en route.

13. b. Use of a helmet can protect the rider against head injury, but not against spinal injury. Leather clothing is helpful in reducing the amount of soft tissue injury. Because the energy of the accident is mostly absorbed into the rider, severe trauma is noted even with low-speed crashes.

14. a. Positive Battle's sign is noted as discoloration of the mastoid area behind the ear. It is an indication that blood has collected there following a basal skull fracture. Periorbital ecchymosis (raccoon's eyes) is noted with facial and orbital trauma and fractures. Subarachnoid bleeding may have no external manifestations or signs.

15. b. The symptoms are indicative of a massforming lesion in the head, such as an epidural or subdural hematoma. When a patient has a simple concussion, the patient's mental status will continue to improve with time.

16. c. The score is 8: two points for eye opening, four points for motor response, and two points for speech.

17. b. These signs and symptoms indicate tension pneumothorax.

18. b. According to the rule of nines for pediatric injuries, the front or back of the trunk each represents 18% of the body surface and the front of one arm represents 4.5% (the entire arm counts for 9%).

19. c. Using the Revised Trauma Score, 3 points for the GCS, 3 points for the systolic blood pressure, and 3 points for the respiratory rate.

20. b. This choice includes the vital sign changes associated with Cushing's reflex.

21. c. Pulmonary contusion involves bruising of the lung tissue. It is essential not to overload a patient suffering from pulmonary contusion with fluids, as this can quickly lead to pulmonary edema. The patient should be given high-flow oxygen and intubated if necessary. Immobilization on a backboard may be necessary depending on the mechanism of injury. If so, the head of the board may be elevated slightly to improve respiratory effort.

22. b. Stabilization of suspected pelvic fractures indicates the use of the PASG/MAST as a splint. Since the systolic blood pressure is less than 90–100 mmHg, IV fluids should be run wide open and **timed** to a normotensive blood pressure.

23. b. Frank blood in the urine is a strong sign of injury to the kidney. Abdominal tenderness is unlikely since the kidneys are located in the retroperitoneal space. Bruising may provide indirect information about organ involvement, but is not as specific as hematuria. Thirst is not one of the most likely symptoms of kidney injury.

24. c. The goal of prehospital care for patients with PID is to provide comfort. There is no need to perform a vaginal exam or ask any questions regarding sexual contacts.

25. b. A patient will breathe more slowly when asleep than when awake; all the other factors listed increase respiratory rate.

26. c. Compliance refers to how easily air flows into and out of the lungs. If compliance is decreasing, look for the cause by reassessing (with look, auscultate, and feel) the airway and head position, and then looking for signs that the patient is developing a tension pneumothorax. Once you find the cause, try to correct it.

27. d. A pulse oximetry reading around 90% for a patient in a normal atmosphere indicates that severe hypoxia is present. It corresponds to a PaO_2 reading of around 60 mmHg. Normal PaO_2 is between 80 and 100 mmHg. Normal pulse oximetry readings are from 93% to 100%, with 93–95% considered the lower end of normal.

28. a. Magill forceps are used to remove an obstructing foreign body that is visible during laryngoscopy after abdominal thrusts have been unsuccessful.

29. b. When the fetus is close to the entrance of the birth canal, the head presses down on the internal anal sphincter, resulting in the urge to have a bowel movement. Painful uterine contractions can start well in advance of physical delivery.

30. d. Air leak over the trachea may be the sign of an improperly inflated cuff, ruling out choice **a.** Right-side-only breath sounds are a sign of right mainstem intubation, ruling out choice **b.** Bilateral chest wall expansion is a normal finding, ruling out choice **c.** The findings in choice **d** point to the need to have a good baseline assessment of lung sounds and respiratory status prior to performing any interventions.

31. b. Rapid onset, crackles, accessory muscle use, and dyspnea are classic symptoms for a patient with acute pulmonary edema.

32. d. Morphine sulfate would be an appropriate treatment for acute pulmonary edema. It increases peripheral venous capacitance and decreases venous return, improving ventilation and decreasing myocardial oxygen demand.

33. b. Immediate transport is indicated for this patient's condition. Without the intact protective amniotic sac, the fetus is at risk of becoming infected.

34. d. Albuterol is a beta-agonist that is used to cause bronchodilation in patients with asthma and other respiratory emergencies. Aminophylline is a methylxanthine in the same class as theophylline. Ipratropium is an anticholinergic bronchodilator. Labetalol is an alpha and beta adrenergic blocker.

35. a. Closed pneumothorax occurs when air enters the pleural space from an interior wound. An open pneumothrax occurs when the chest wall is open so that air can enter directly into the chest from the outside. A tension pneumothorax develops when a simple pneumothorax becomes large enough to cause pressure and structural changes within the chest.

36. d. Stridor, a sound made during inspiration, is associated with croup and upper-airway obstruction.

37. a. A baby in single-limb presentation is considered nondeliverable vaginally and requires a rapid cesarean section to be successfully delivered. Rapid transport is indicated.

38. b. Patients with emphysema or chronic bronchitis benefit from administration of low-flow oxygen and constant monitoring.

39. a. As a bronchodilator, epinephrine 1:1,000 may be indicated in younger (< 35 years old) asthma patients.

40. c. A patient who is conscious and breathing over 30 times per minute is classified as immediate. There is no need to check for the presence or rate of the pulse. While she may need oxygen therapy, now is not the time to apply it.

41. a. The inspiratory stridor most likely indicates an edematous crushed or torn trachea.

42. c. This patient's symptoms indicate subcutaneous emphysema.

43. b. It will be difficult to determine the actual extent of injury, so the least invasive airway technique is appropriate. Monitor vital signs and pulse oximetry readings to determine if perfusion is adequate.

44. a. Given the circumstances, not enough personnel are available to restrain this patient if he becomes violent. Conducting a hands-on assessment may not be possible given the state of the patient's behavior. Constantly being aware of your surroundings will provide the greatest level of safety.

45. d. Aeromedical transport offers the advantage of rapid transport to specialized facilities such as the Level I Trauma Center. Given the amount of time needed to extricate the patient, coupled with the time to transport the patient to either the closest hospital or the trauma center by ground, flying the patient directly to the trauma center is most appropriate.

46. c. The first sign of laryngeal edema usually is a hoarse voice.

47. d. Patients with emphysema have a loss of elasticity in the alveoli due to prolonged insult. Bleb formation results in the decreased ability of the alveoli to expand and contract and an overall decreased surface area of the lungs. Ruptured blebs do not result in lung deflation.

48. c. This patient is exhibiting the classic signs and symptoms of congestive heart failure. His history of AMI indicates that he may have permanent damage to the heart and raises the possibility that he is now having an acute episode of failure.

49. d. Oxygen, morphine, nitroglycerin, and furosemide are all used in the treatment of CHF patients.

50. b. Paroxysmal nocturnal dyspnea (PND), dyspnea upon exertion, and increased dyspnea are all signs of worsening CHF.

51. b. Choices **a**, **c**, and **d** indicate priorities for managing this patient.

52. d. Increased ventilatory pressures assist in driving off some of the pulmonary edema.

53. d. Choices **a**, **b**, and **c** are all typically associated with CHF; syncope is not.

54. a. Isotonic solutions such as lactated Ringer's or normal saline have electrolyte compositions similar to that of blood plasma, although they lack the large protein molecules found within blood.

55. c. Managing the patient's injury is the first priority of the EMS provider. Any statements made by the patient should be recorded as possible evidence of the crime.

56. a. A sprain is a partial tearing of a ligament caused by a sudden twisting or stretching of a joint beyond its normal range of motion. It results in swelling and discoloration caused by bleeding into the tissue. A strain is an injury to the muscle or tendon and usually does not result in discoloration. A dislocation occurs when the normal articulation of two bones is disrupted. Arthritis is inflammation of joints characterized by pain and swelling but does not result in discoloration.

57. b. Morphine relieves pain, decreases venous return, and reduces the oxygen demand of the myocardium.

58. c. Left-sided heart failure with pulmonary edema is often associated with PND. PND manifests as difficulty breathing when the patient lies flat. As the condition worsens, many patients will report the need to sleep sitting up in a recliner.

59. b. As the tip of the nasotracheal tube reaches the glottic opening, you should hear the respiratory effort of the patient. Insertion of the tube past the vocal cords is timed to the inhalation phase in order to minimize resistance against the tube itself.

60. c. The preferred field treatment is transcutaneous pacing. Definitive treatment is pacemaker insertion. Drug therapy indicated for this patient is aimed at increasing cardiac output by improving contractility, force of contractions, or increasing rate.

61. a. Treat the patient for shock and transport rapidly. Do not palpate the abdomen. Consider permissive reduction of blood pressure and heart rate using beta blockers. This reduction can help to prevent the aneurysm from dissecting during transport.

62. b. This patient needs immediate oxygenation and ventilation. Using a bag-valve mask will accomplish this task most effectively.

63. d. PSVTs (paroxysmal supraventricular tachycardia) may be managed by vagal maneuvers, such as the Valsalva maneuver or ice-water immersion.

64. b. The length of a normal P-R interval is 0.12–0.20 seconds, or 3–5 small boxes on the ECG strip.

65. b. The high-pitched whistling noise and cyanosis indicates the patient is suffering from an airway obstruction. Back blows and chest thrusts are performed only on infants. Since the patient is unresponsive, your immediate step should be to start CPR. For unresponsive victims suspected of having an airway obstruction, you should begin CPR, but look in the mouth to see if you visualize the object prior to each ventilation attempt. Abdominal thrusts are performed only on conscious choking victims.

66. d. Stridor indicates an upper-airway obstruction, in this case most likely from an allergic reaction. A patient suffering from a CVA would have an altered mental status but would not have stridor. A patient with emphysema would exhibit difficulty breathing with wheezing and rhonchi. A patient with asthma will exhibit wheezing respirations.

67. c. Patients with ventricular dysrhythmias often manifest lengthened and bizarre QRS complexes.

68. a. Treatment for both conditions consists of immediate defibrillation; continued treatment includes CPR and drugs. Additional therapy depends on if a normal rhythm is initiated.

69. a. These are the classic signs and symptoms of right-side heart failure.

70. a. The position of comfort for most people having trouble breathing is sitting; however, this patient may have low blood pressure, possibly due to a cardiac emergency. In this case, it would be important to ensure that her blood pressure is adequate to support a sudden change in body position.

71. d. Anxiety and pain can increase the heart rate and, therefore, the oxygen demand of the myocardium.

72. b. Dopamine is a potent sympathomimetic agent and, in cases of cardiogenic shock, may be used to increase cardiac output.

73. a. The question does not provide any indication of a tension pneumothorax. A pulmonary contusion or cardiac tamponade should not affect lung sounds.

74. b. Intramuscular injections can injure muscle tissues, causing the release of enzymes that may mask the cardiac enzymes that confirm a diagnosis of MI.

75. b. A patient with angina whose pain does not respond to nitroglycerin is most likely suffering from an AMI and should be transported without delay.

76. a. COPD patients can no longer rely upon normal regulatory mechanisms to control their respirations. The hypoxic drive measures for low levels of oxygen in the bloodstream to increase respiratory rate.

77. a. Lidocaine is the first drug used to treat malignant PVCs or nonmalignant PVCs in patients who are symptomatic or who have a history of cardiac disease. Bretylium is no longer available commercially. Procainamide and magnesium sulfate are used if v-fib or v-tach develops; they also may be used to treat PVCs after a trial of lidocaine has been unsuccessful.

78. b. If the trach tube has been dislodged, it may not be easy to reinsert, so rest it in its original position. Placing an endotracheal tube into the stoma and inflating the cuff will help rapidly establish a patient's airway.

79. b. Dilated pupils, hyperactivity, tachycardia, and hypertension are classic signs of cocaine use. Narcotic use would result in lethargy, stupor, and respiratory depression.

80. a. Transport is the only other treatment required for this patient. Be prepared to provide respiratory support if needed. Naloxone is used with narcotic ingestion to restore respirations and is not indicated for this patient. Activated charcoal and ipecac are indicated for poisoning or overdose via the oral route. This patient was reported to have inhaled (smoked) something that appears to be a stimulant.

81. c. Dysrhythmias and seizures are both serious possible complications of stimulation effects from cocaine use.

82. b. This patient appears to be experiencing acute pulmonary edema. Of the choices provided, choice **b** has both the correct doses and routes of the indicated medications.

83. b. Reduced pumping capacity of the right ventricle causes blood flow to back up into the systemic vascular system, causing congestion as evidenced by the pedal edema and jugular venous distention (JVD). Lung fields that are past the cardiac insufficiency remain free from fluid.

84. c. The neutral position, or position of function, for the hand is achieved by using a gauze roller bandage (or similar material) placed inside the palm with the fingers curled around it. The hand, wrist, and forearm should then be splinted with a board, wire ladder, or vacuum-type splint.

85. a. Do not allow the severed digit to get wet because the tissues will begin to draw in the hypotonic fluid and will swell up, which may make reimplantation impossible. The cold environment will help reduce oxygen demand by the cells of the severed digit and will help keep it viable longer.

86. d. Pit viper envenomation is generally very painful. Little or no pain is characteristic of coral snake (neurotoxic) envenomation.

87. b. Brush away as much of the lime as possible, then flood the burned area with water. Immersing the injured limb in water keeps the patient in contact with the chemical agent. Neutralizing chemicals are generally not recommended because the use of one chemical to neutralize another usually results in the release of heat and the formation of a third chemical.

88. a. Hypoglycemia develops in patients with diabetes when they take too much insulin or exercise too much for the amount of food they eat.

89. b. Central neurogenic hyperventilation is characterized by rapid, deep, noisy breathing and is associated with lesions of the central nervous system. Cheyne-Stokes respiration is the pattern commonly seen with diabetic emergencies.

90. b. *Do not resuscitate* is not the same as *do not treat*. Under these conditions, management of the condition is warranted, and choice **b** is the appropriate course of action.

91. a. The first priority for patients with altered mental status of unknown cause is a blood glucose determination to rule out hypoglycemia as a potential cause.

92. d. For a patient in status epilepticus, treatment consists of establishing an IV, monitoring cardiac rhythm, and administering diazepam to stop the seizures.

93. a. This is the standard adult dosage and route for a patient with severe anaphylaxis. Services may recommend the use of 1:1,000 instead 1:10,000.

94. d. The very young, the very old, those undernourished, and those with chronic illness are all predisposed to heat illnesses for a variety of reasons.

95. d. Bradycardia in a child is an ominous sign of a hypoxic brain.

96. c. Provide oxygen at 100% concentration and intubate if the patient is not breathing spontaneously.

97. c. The purpose of the interview is to calm the patient and to obtain as much information as possible, not to tell the patient what you think. There is a time to reorient patients to reality, but first you must work to calm them down and gain their trust.

98. c. The lumbar spine will be most impacted from an unevenly distributed load; the cervical spine is also at risk for injury, although such injuries are less likely.

99. a. The patient's presentation suggests a pulmonary embolism is the likely cause. The other conditions are not normally associated with sudden syncope, and adventitious lung sounds, like crackles or wheezes, should be evident, unlike the patient's clear ones.

100. c. Unusual respiratory patterns indicate the possibility of brain stem injury and call for rapid transport of the patient. Hyperventilation should be used only when you strongly suspect herniation is occurring. It is not indicated for the routine treatment of increasing ICP. You should ventilate the patient at a normal rate with 100% oxygen.

101. b. Medical direction should be sought if at all possible for any suspected substance-abuse patient refusing treatment or transport. It is not advisable to allow the patient to sign a refusal form when it is obvious that the patient is in need of medical attention. Because you are required to be an advocate for the patient, it is not advisable to transport someone against the patient's will, even if you suspect impairment due to drug or alcohol use. Treating the patient and then leaving the scene without transport leaves you open to legal liability and a possible charge of abandonment.

102. c. It is important in this situation to make a complete documentation of the patient's refusal to accept treatment. Documentation should include the steps you took to convince the patient to seek medical attention, the potential consequences of the patient's refusal, and your assessment findings.

103. b. This choice gives the most appropriate treatment protocol for this patient. Because the patient is unconscious, the patient may be treated under implied consent. Treatment in this case is aimed at ruling out the most treatable cause for coma—diabetes.

104. b. While it is possible that he could have a pulmonary embolism, the more likely culprit is a simple pneumothorax. He has few risk factors for a PE, and lung sounds usually remain present unless a large area of pulmonary tissue is not perfused for some period of time.

105. a. The patient is experiencing an unstable atrial fibrillation. He is hypotensive and tachypneic. In this situation, it is imperative to capture the atrial rate as soon as possible. The ventricular rate will decrease once the atria are under control.

106. b. A spontaneous pneumothorax occurs when a bleb (cystic lesion on the lobe of the lung) ruptures, allowing air to enter the pleural space from within the lung. It usually occurs in otherwise healthy individuals ages 20 to 40. They are usually well tolerated and occupy less than 20% of a lung.

107. a. The best place to assess for cyanosis in an infant or child is the oral mucosa, lips, or tongue. Nail beds of an infant may not be an accurate indicator of central circulation status even when they appear cyanotic.

108. a. Give a severely dehydrated child an initial bolus of 20 mL/kg of normal saline or Ringer's solution. Reassess for response and repeat with 10 or 20 mL/kg boluses as long as the child continues to improve and you do not detect any signs of fluid overload.

109. a. In this situation, the first step would be to examine the patient for crowning to determine if you need to assist with delivery on the scene or if you can attempt to transport her.

110. a. The protruding umbilical cord is known as a prolapsed cord.

111. d. Choices **a**, **b**, and **c** are all appropriate treatment options for this patient. If you opt to position the patient for transport, you should place her in the left-lateral recumbent position to improve uterine blood flow and return.

112. a. The umbilical vein, found within the umbilical cord, provides oxygenated blood to the infant. The vein is large enough for you to feel the pulsations as blood flows from the placenta to the fetus. If the cord cools down, an arterial vasospasm may occur, resulting in the cessation of blood flow to the infant, but the cord temperature does not correlate to the infant's temperature, ruling out choice **b**. The umbilical cord has various color gradations from red to purplish and the relationship between color and oxygen level is difficult to determine, ruling out choice **c**. Pulse oximetry is not appropriate for fetal monitoring in the method described, ruling out choice **d**.

113. c. G4 P3 refers to a woman who has been pregnant four times and delivered three live infants.

114. c. *Effacement* refers to the stretching and thinning of the cervix, which occurs during the first stage of normal labor.

115. a. These are the signs and symptoms of abruptio placentae, or premature separation of the placenta.

116. b. Patients with preeclampsia (or toxemia of pregnancy) manifest all the signs and symptoms of hypertensive disorders of pregnancy except seizures. Once the patient begins to experience seizures, the condition has changed from preeclampsia to eclampsia.

117. c. The third stage of labor begins with the birth of the fetus and ends with the delivery of the placenta.

118. d. Clamp the cord in two places, approximately 5 cm apart, and cut the cord between the clamps. Generally, you want to place the first clamp several (5–7) cm away from the infant.

119. d. Heart rate at birth is normally 150–180 beats per minute, slowing to 130–140 within a few minutes.

120. d. Chest compressions are required when a newborn's heart rate is less than 60, or between 60 and 80 after 30 seconds of positive-pressure ventilation. Remember to perform each intervention for approximately 30 seconds, then reassess for the need to continue resuscitation.

121. b. The umbilical vein, located in the umbilical cord, is used for this purpose. If the cord is left untreated at the hospital, it may be cannulated for a week or even longer. It enters immediately into the hepatic circulation.

122. d. Fever-induced seizures are common in young children with only minor illnesses. Once a child has a febrile seizure, he or she is prone to repeat episodes, which can occur at lower temperatures than the first seizure.

123. a. Increased body temperature, tachycardia, and tachypnea are common in a child who is recently postictal from febrile seizures.

124. c. Oxygen, an IV, and transport is an appropriate treatment for this patient. Remove excess clothing from the patient to passively cool him or her, but do not allow the patient to get chilled. Sponge the child with room temperature water if the temperature is excessively high. Never use alcohol on the skin as a cooling agent. Alcohol can be absorbed directly through the skin.

125. b. This patient is in cardiac arrest with a cardiac rhythm characteristic of ventricular tachycardia (v-tach). Because the patient has renal failure, the initial approach should consist of rapid defibrillation and antidysrhythmics. All such patients should be assumed to be hyperkalemic and should be treated with a combination of sodium bicarbonate and calcium gluconate, which work together to move the potassium into cells and out of the bloodstream.

126. c. The patient's rapid onset reduces the possibility of pneumonia. Patients with emphysema are prone to experiencing a simple pneumothorax. No information indicates any other medical condition such as asthma or chronic bronchitis.

127. b. A type II ambulance is an integral unit consisting of a standard van, usually with a raised roof.

128. d. The living will and DNR order are both examples of legal documents called advanced directives. They specify the kind of healthcare a person does and does not want to receive in the event of their imminent death. A durable power of attorney does not specify treatment—it allows another to make healthcare decisions for an individual.

129. c. In most states, consent for treatment must be obtained from all patients who are 18 years old or older. This can be modified in situations of extenuating circumstances, such as when an underage minor is pregnant or has legal custody of a minor child in the patient's care.

130. d. Snoring respirations are indicative of an airway issue and should be corrected before further assessment is completed.

131. c. The GCS for this patient is 12: three points for opening her eyes to verbal stimuli, five points for localizing pain, and four points for speaking clearly although her thought process is confused.

132. a. The first paramedic unit to arrive at the scene of a mass-casualty incident would immediately assume command and transmit a report to dispatch, alerting them to the need for more units. As other units begin to arrive, they may be detailed to perform triage or some other duty.

133. c. The respiratory rate is too slow and must be corrected immediately with ventilatory assistance.

134. d. In the START system, a patient with respirations greater than 30 per minute would receive immediate attention. Patient **a** would not receive any care beyond the initial opening of the airway. Patients **b** and **c** would receive additional assessment before treatment.

135. d. Bulimia and anorexia nervosa are both common eating disorders. They both have similar features such as misperceptions of body image. Bulimia involves binge eating followed by self-induced vomiting.

136. a. All the others do not have critical mechanisms, so they should not receive rapid transportation.

137. a. Commonly accepted infection-control guidelines call for all personnel to wear masks and protective eyewear for any procedure that carries the risk of splashing of blood, vomitus, or other fluids.

138. c. Accidental needle sticks are the most common source of work-related HIV and hepatitis B infections in healthcare workers.

139. d. Because cardiac disease is so common, you should administer medications commonly prescribed for other types of emergencies with extreme caution.

140. b. Toddlers can often be reassured by being allowed to handle unfamiliar objects. They will not understand detailed explanations and should not be allowed to disassemble equipment.

141. a. Battle's sign is the black-and-blue discoloration just behind the ears. Periorbital ecchymosis is black-and-blue discoloration around the eyes, also known as raccoon eyes. Both are classic signs of a basilar skull fracture.

142. c. Women attempt suicide more often, but men are more successful at it. Also, men choose more deadly means. About 60% of the people who successfully commit suicide have a history of previous attempts.

143. c. A multiplex system allows for a two-way conversation and simultaneous transmission of telemetry readings.

144. b. The rhythm is coarse ventricular fibrillation.

145. d. The ST segment elevation in leads I, AVL, V5, and V6 are indicative of a lateral wall myocardial infarction.

146. c. This patient's chest pain is most likely due to the supraventricular tachycardia. The patient's presentation and vital signs indicate he is compensating well enough to start with the least invasive treatment, vagal maneuvers, progress to 3 doses of adenosine, and finally perform synchronized cardioversion.

147. c. The rhythm is sinus tachycardia. The rate is greater than 100 and there is a p wave for each QRS, which are narrow.

148. a. The delta wave is an indicator of Wolff-Parkinson-White syndrome. A J wave is indicative of hypothermia. Hyperkalemia is indicated by peaked T waves. Hypokalemia is indicated by a U wave that can cause the QRS complexes to appear widened.

149. d. Apart from time, there is no reversal agent for succinylcholine.

150. b. Normal physiologic PEEP is between 3–5 cm H_2O.

Scoring

Evaluate how you did on this practice exam by first finding the number of questions you answered correctly. Only the number of correct answers is important—questions you skipped or answered incorrectly do not count against your score. Your goal should be a score greater than 80%. The NREMT exam is now computer adaptive and therefore there is no minimum score, just a measure of competency.

Use your scores in conjunction with the LearningExpress Test Preparation System in Chapter 2 of this book to help devise a study plan. You should plan to spend more time on the topics that correspond to the questions you found hardest, and less time on the topics in which you performed well.

Much more important than your overall score, for now, is how you did on each of the topics tested by the exam. You need to diagnose your strengths and weaknesses so that you can concentrate your efforts as you prepare. The question types are mixed in the practice exam, so in order to tell where your strengths and weaknesses lie, you will need to compare your answer sheet with the following table that shows the topic for each question.

PARAMEDIC PRACTICE EXAM 2 DIAGNOSTIC SCORING CHART

TOPIC	QUESTION #
Airway, Respiration, and Ventilation	2, 25, 26, 27, 28, 30, 36, 38, 41, 42, 43, 46, 47, 59, 62, 65, 70, 76, 78, 95, 99, 106, 107, 126, 130, 133, 150
Cardiology and Resuscitation	31, 32, 48, 49, 50, 51, 52, 53, 57, 58, 60, 63, 64, 67, 68, 69, 71, 74, 75, 77, 82, 83, 105, 120, 121, 125, 139, 144, 145, 146, 147, 148
Trauma	1, 4, 5, 6, 12, 13, 14, 15, 16, 17, 18, 19, 20, 21, 22, 23, 35, 56, 73, 84, 85, 86, 87, 89, 100, 131, 136, 141
Medical/Obstetrics/Gynecology	8, 9, 10, 11, 24, 29, 33, 37, 61, 66, 79, 80, 81, 88, 91, 92, 93, 94, 96, 97, 103, 104, 108, 109, 110, 111, 112, 113, 114, 115, 116, 117, 118, 119, 122, 123, 124, 135, 142
EMS Operations	3, 7, 34, 39, 40, 44, 45, 54, 55, 72, 90, 98, 101, 102, 127, 128, 129, 132, 134, 137, 138, 140, 143, 149

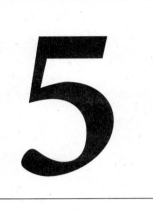

5 ▶ PARAMEDIC PRACTICE EXAM 3

CHAPTER SUMMARY

This is the third of five practice exams in this book based on the NREMT EMT-Paramedic/Paramedic written exam. Use this test to identify which types of questions are still giving you problems.

You are now becoming very familiar with the format of the NREMT EMT-Paramedic/Paramedic exam. Your practice test-taking experience will help you most if you have created a situation that closely mirrors the day of the official test.

For this third exam, simulate a real test. Find a quiet place where you will not be disturbed. Have with you two sharpened pencils and a good eraser. Complete the test in one sitting, setting a timer or a stopwatch. You should have plenty of time to answer all of the questions when you take the real exam, but you want to practice working quickly without rushing.

The answer sheet you should use is on the next page. Following the exam is an answer key that will help you see where you need to concentrate further study. When you have finished the exam and scored it, turn to the diagnostic scoring chart at the end of the chapter to see which areas of the exam give you the most trouble. Then you will know which parts of your textbook to concentrate on before you take the fourth exam.

1.	ⓐ	ⓑ	ⓒ	ⓓ		51.	ⓐ	ⓑ	ⓒ	ⓓ		101.	ⓐ	ⓑ	ⓒ	ⓓ
2.	ⓐ	ⓑ	ⓒ	ⓓ		52.	ⓐ	ⓑ	ⓒ	ⓓ		102.	ⓐ	ⓑ	ⓒ	ⓓ
3.	ⓐ	ⓑ	ⓒ	ⓓ		53.	ⓐ	ⓑ	ⓒ	ⓓ		103.	ⓐ	ⓑ	ⓒ	ⓓ
4.	ⓐ	ⓑ	ⓒ	ⓓ		54.	ⓐ	ⓑ	ⓒ	ⓓ		104.	ⓐ	ⓑ	ⓒ	ⓓ
5.	ⓐ	ⓑ	ⓒ	ⓓ		55.	ⓐ	ⓑ	ⓒ	ⓓ		105.	ⓐ	ⓑ	ⓒ	ⓓ
6.	ⓐ	ⓑ	ⓒ	ⓓ		56.	ⓐ	ⓑ	ⓒ	ⓓ		106.	ⓐ	ⓑ	ⓒ	ⓓ
7.	ⓐ	ⓑ	ⓒ	ⓓ		57.	ⓐ	ⓑ	ⓒ	ⓓ		107.	ⓐ	ⓑ	ⓒ	ⓓ
8.	ⓐ	ⓑ	ⓒ	ⓓ		58.	ⓐ	ⓑ	ⓒ	ⓓ		108.	ⓐ	ⓑ	ⓒ	ⓓ
9.	ⓐ	ⓑ	ⓒ	ⓓ		59.	ⓐ	ⓑ	ⓒ	ⓓ		109.	ⓐ	ⓑ	ⓒ	ⓓ
10.	ⓐ	ⓑ	ⓒ	ⓓ		60.	ⓐ	ⓑ	ⓒ	ⓓ		110.	ⓐ	ⓑ	ⓒ	ⓓ
11.	ⓐ	ⓑ	ⓒ	ⓓ		61.	ⓐ	ⓑ	ⓒ	ⓓ		111.	ⓐ	ⓑ	ⓒ	ⓓ
12.	ⓐ	ⓑ	ⓒ	ⓓ		62.	ⓐ	ⓑ	ⓒ	ⓓ		112.	ⓐ	ⓑ	ⓒ	ⓓ
13.	ⓐ	ⓑ	ⓒ	ⓓ		63.	ⓐ	ⓑ	ⓒ	ⓓ		113.	ⓐ	ⓑ	ⓒ	ⓓ
14.	ⓐ	ⓑ	ⓒ	ⓓ		64.	ⓐ	ⓑ	ⓒ	ⓓ		114.	ⓐ	ⓑ	ⓒ	ⓓ
15.	ⓐ	ⓑ	ⓒ	ⓓ		65.	ⓐ	ⓑ	ⓒ	ⓓ		115.	ⓐ	ⓑ	ⓒ	ⓓ
16.	ⓐ	ⓑ	ⓒ	ⓓ		66.	ⓐ	ⓑ	ⓒ	ⓓ		116.	ⓐ	ⓑ	ⓒ	ⓓ
17.	ⓐ	ⓑ	ⓒ	ⓓ		67.	ⓐ	ⓑ	ⓒ	ⓓ		117.	ⓐ	ⓑ	ⓒ	ⓓ
18.	ⓐ	ⓑ	ⓒ	ⓓ		68.	ⓐ	ⓑ	ⓒ	ⓓ		118.	ⓐ	ⓑ	ⓒ	ⓓ
19.	ⓐ	ⓑ	ⓒ	ⓓ		69.	ⓐ	ⓑ	ⓒ	ⓓ		119.	ⓐ	ⓑ	ⓒ	ⓓ
20.	ⓐ	ⓑ	ⓒ	ⓓ		70.	ⓐ	ⓑ	ⓒ	ⓓ		120.	ⓐ	ⓑ	ⓒ	ⓓ
21.	ⓐ	ⓑ	ⓒ	ⓓ		71.	ⓐ	ⓑ	ⓒ	ⓓ		121.	ⓐ	ⓑ	ⓒ	ⓓ
22.	ⓐ	ⓑ	ⓒ	ⓓ		72.	ⓐ	ⓑ	ⓒ	ⓓ		122.	ⓐ	ⓑ	ⓒ	ⓓ
23.	ⓐ	ⓑ	ⓒ	ⓓ		73.	ⓐ	ⓑ	ⓒ	ⓓ		123.	ⓐ	ⓑ	ⓒ	ⓓ
24.	ⓐ	ⓑ	ⓒ	ⓓ		74.	ⓐ	ⓑ	ⓒ	ⓓ		124.	ⓐ	ⓑ	ⓒ	ⓓ
25.	ⓐ	ⓑ	ⓒ	ⓓ		75.	ⓐ	ⓑ	ⓒ	ⓓ		125.	ⓐ	ⓑ	ⓒ	ⓓ
26.	ⓐ	ⓑ	ⓒ	ⓓ		76.	ⓐ	ⓑ	ⓒ	ⓓ		126.	ⓐ	ⓑ	ⓒ	ⓓ
27.	ⓐ	ⓑ	ⓒ	ⓓ		77.	ⓐ	ⓑ	ⓒ	ⓓ		127.	ⓐ	ⓑ	ⓒ	ⓓ
28.	ⓐ	ⓑ	ⓒ	ⓓ		78.	ⓐ	ⓑ	ⓒ	ⓓ		128.	ⓐ	ⓑ	ⓒ	ⓓ
29.	ⓐ	ⓑ	ⓒ	ⓓ		79.	ⓐ	ⓑ	ⓒ	ⓓ		129.	ⓐ	ⓑ	ⓒ	ⓓ
30.	ⓐ	ⓑ	ⓒ	ⓓ		80.	ⓐ	ⓑ	ⓒ	ⓓ		130.	ⓐ	ⓑ	ⓒ	ⓓ
31.	ⓐ	ⓑ	ⓒ	ⓓ		81.	ⓐ	ⓑ	ⓒ	ⓓ		131.	ⓐ	ⓑ	ⓒ	ⓓ
32.	ⓐ	ⓑ	ⓒ	ⓓ		82.	ⓐ	ⓑ	ⓒ	ⓓ		132.	ⓐ	ⓑ	ⓒ	ⓓ
33.	ⓐ	ⓑ	ⓒ	ⓓ		83.	ⓐ	ⓑ	ⓒ	ⓓ		133.	ⓐ	ⓑ	ⓒ	ⓓ
34.	ⓐ	ⓑ	ⓒ	ⓓ		84.	ⓐ	ⓑ	ⓒ	ⓓ		134.	ⓐ	ⓑ	ⓒ	ⓓ
35.	ⓐ	ⓑ	ⓒ	ⓓ		85.	ⓐ	ⓑ	ⓒ	ⓓ		135.	ⓐ	ⓑ	ⓒ	ⓓ
36.	ⓐ	ⓑ	ⓒ	ⓓ		86.	ⓐ	ⓑ	ⓒ	ⓓ		136.	ⓐ	ⓑ	ⓒ	ⓓ
37.	ⓐ	ⓑ	ⓒ	ⓓ		87.	ⓐ	ⓑ	ⓒ	ⓓ		137.	ⓐ	ⓑ	ⓒ	ⓓ
38.	ⓐ	ⓑ	ⓒ	ⓓ		88.	ⓐ	ⓑ	ⓒ	ⓓ		138.	ⓐ	ⓑ	ⓒ	ⓓ
39.	ⓐ	ⓑ	ⓒ	ⓓ		89.	ⓐ	ⓑ	ⓒ	ⓓ		139.	ⓐ	ⓑ	ⓒ	ⓓ
40.	ⓐ	ⓑ	ⓒ	ⓓ		90.	ⓐ	ⓑ	ⓒ	ⓓ		140.	ⓐ	ⓑ	ⓒ	ⓓ
41.	ⓐ	ⓑ	ⓒ	ⓓ		91.	ⓐ	ⓑ	ⓒ	ⓓ		141.	ⓐ	ⓑ	ⓒ	ⓓ
42.	ⓐ	ⓑ	ⓒ	ⓓ		92.	ⓐ	ⓑ	ⓒ	ⓓ		142.	ⓐ	ⓑ	ⓒ	ⓓ
43.	ⓐ	ⓑ	ⓒ	ⓓ		93.	ⓐ	ⓑ	ⓒ	ⓓ		143.	ⓐ	ⓑ	ⓒ	ⓓ
44.	ⓐ	ⓑ	ⓒ	ⓓ		94.	ⓐ	ⓑ	ⓒ	ⓓ		144.	ⓐ	ⓑ	ⓒ	ⓓ
45.	ⓐ	ⓑ	ⓒ	ⓓ		95.	ⓐ	ⓑ	ⓒ	ⓓ		145.	ⓐ	ⓑ	ⓒ	ⓓ
46.	ⓐ	ⓑ	ⓒ	ⓓ		96.	ⓐ	ⓑ	ⓒ	ⓓ		146.	ⓐ	ⓑ	ⓒ	ⓓ
47.	ⓐ	ⓑ	ⓒ	ⓓ		97.	ⓐ	ⓑ	ⓒ	ⓓ		147.	ⓐ	ⓑ	ⓒ	ⓓ
48.	ⓐ	ⓑ	ⓒ	ⓓ		98.	ⓐ	ⓑ	ⓒ	ⓓ		148.	ⓐ	ⓑ	ⓒ	ⓓ
49.	ⓐ	ⓑ	ⓒ	ⓓ		99.	ⓐ	ⓑ	ⓒ	ⓓ		149.	ⓐ	ⓑ	ⓒ	ⓓ
50.	ⓐ	ⓑ	ⓒ	ⓓ		100.	ⓐ	ⓑ	ⓒ	ⓓ		150.	ⓐ	ⓑ	ⓒ	ⓓ

Paramedic Exam 3

1. Which organs are contained in the right upper quadrant of the abdomen?
   a. spleen, tail of pancreas, stomach, left kidney, and part of the colon
   b. liver, gall bladder, head of the pancreas, part of the duodenum, and part of the colon
   c. appendix, ascending colon, small intestine, right ovary, and fallopian tube
   d. small intestine, descending colon, left ovary, and fallopian tube

2. Chest pain associated with stable angina may be caused by which of the following?
   a. a buildup of lactic acid and CO_2
   b. an occluded coronary artery
   c. cardiac dysrhythmias
   d. cardiac cell death

3. Your patient is a 65-year-old female complaining of chest pressure. The ECG shows a wide complex tachycardia at a rate of 200 beats per minute. The patient's vital signs are P 200 BPM, RR 26 breaths per minute, and BP 90/60 mmHg. Which of the following is the best treatment for this patient?
   a. lidocaine 0.5–1.0 mg/kg IVP
   b. synchronized cardioversion at 100 joules
   c. defibrillation at 200 joules
   d. amiodarone 150 mg IVP, pushed slowly

4. To what does pulse pressure refer?
   a. diastolic blood pressure reading × the systolic reading
   b. systolic × the diastolic blood pressure reading
   c. difference between the systolic and diastolic readings
   d. systolic blood pressure as measured by a Doppler device

5. A 56-year-old male experienced a syncopal episode and is now complaining of intense chest pressure. His vital signs are RR 26 breaths per minute, P 110 BPM, and BP 80/64 mmHg. Crackles can be auscultated in both lower lung fields. Which of the following conditions best defines the patient's presentation?
   a. acute pulmonary embolism
   b. cardiogenic shock
   c. cardiac arrest
   d. malignant hypotension

6. An elderly male is complaining of a sudden onset of severe pain in his right leg. The affected extremity is cool to the touch and pale. The temperature and pulse in the patient's left leg is normal. You suspect which of the following?
   a. varicose arteries
   b. arterial occlusion
   c. pulmonary embolism
   d. deep-vein thrombosis

Answer questions 7–9 based on the following information.

You arrive at a golf course to find a 45-year-old male unconscious and responsive to pain only with movement. The patient was struck in the head by a golf ball traveling at high velocity. His eyes are closed; pupil examination reveals his left pupil is 2 mm, and the right is 8 mm and not reactive to light. This patient moves upper extremities to localized pain and moves lower extremities spontaneously. He is breathing full deep respirations at a rate of 24 per minute.

7. You would expect the vital signs of this patient generally to follow which of the following groupings?
   a. RR increased, HR decreased, BP decreased
   b. RR irregular, HR decreased, BP increased
   c. RR decreased, HR decreased, BP decreased
   d. RR irregular, HR increased, BP increased

8. Treatment of this patient would include which of the following?
   a. spinal immobilization to a long board with cervical collar
   b. IV fluid boluses titrated to a systolic BP of 100–110 mmHg
   c. opening the patient's airway using the head-tilt/chin-lift technique
   d. placing the patient in the sniffing position to facilitate airflow

9. A patient with a closed head injury should be closely monitored for all EXCEPT which one of the following?
   a. hypovolemic shock
   b. respiratory alkalosis
   c. hypoxic seizures
   d. hemopneumothorax

10. Your patient, a car accident victim, complains of seeing "a dark curtain" in front of one eye. What should you suspect?
   a. optic nerve damage
   b. retinal detachment
   c. orbital fracture
   d. subconjunctival hemorrhage

11. Treatment for a patient in cardiogenic shock who is complaining of chest pressure should include which of the following?
   a. adenosine IV push
   b. furosemide IV push
   c. dopamine infusion
   d. nitroglycerin SL

12. Signs and symptoms of traumatic asphyxia include
   a. paradoxical chest motion, pain on inspiration, and increased respiratory rate.
   b. dyspnea, bloodshot eyes, distended neck veins, and a cyanotic upper body.
   c. agitation, air hunger, distended neck veins, shock, and tracheal displacement.
   d. shock, cyanosis, absent breath sounds over one lobe, and flat neck veins.

13. An adult patient has burns covering her head and upper back. Using the rule of nines, this patient's burns cover what percentage of her body surface area?
   a. 9%
   b. 18%
   c. 27%
   d. 36%

14. How would you classify a burn that is pearly white and almost painless?
   a. first-degree burn
   b. second-degree burn
   c. third-degree burn
   d. chemical burn

15. Which of the following conditions indicates the need for rapid transport?
   a. isolated penetrating trauma by a knife in the upper forearm
   b. a pedestrian struck by a motor vehicle traveling about 10 mph
   c. first-degree and second-degree burns to the anterior chest
   d. pulse rate 130 BPM; blood pressure 90/60 mmHg; and respiratory rate 36 breaths per minute

16. What is the Glasgow Coma Scale score for a patient who opens her eyes in response to pain, speaks incomprehensibly, and withdraws in response to pain?
- **a.** 6
- **b.** 7
- **c.** 8
- **d.** 9

17 Your patient is a 23-year-old man who complains of abdominal pain. The patient states that the pain began suddenly and was originally located only in the area around the umbilicus. However, it has now moved to the right lower quadrant. The patient also complains of nausea and vomiting, and he has a fever of 102°F. Examination displays rebound tenderness. What condition should you suspect?
- **a.** diverticulitis
- **b.** gastritis
- **c.** peptic ulcer
- **d.** appendicitis

18. A 42-year-old male complains of sudden, intense pain that is centered in his lower back. He is pale, cool, and diaphoretic, especially below the level of his umbilicus. He is tachycardic and hypotensive. Which of the following conditions best describes the patient presentation?
- **a.** myocardial infarction
- **b.** abdominal aortic aneurysm
- **c.** pancreatitis
- **d.** kidney stones

19. Your patient is a 76-year-old male who is complaining of malaise. He has no medical history and takes no medications. His blood pressure is 112/70 mmHg, pulse is 60 BPM and irregular, respirations 20 breaths per minute, lungs are clear and equal bilaterally, and skin is warm and dry. Figure 5.1 depicts his ECG. Prehospital management of this patient includes
- **a.** oxygen and monitoring only.
- **b.** oxygen and IV atropine.
- **c.** oxygen and transcutaneous pacing.
- **d.** oxygen, atropine, and transcutaneous pacing.

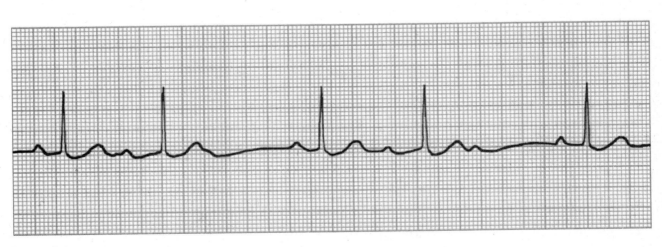

Figure 5.1

20. Of what does the initial symptom of infection with HIV primarily consist?
a. mild fatigue and fever
b. encephalopathy
c. Kaposi's sarcoma
d. Pneumocystis carinii

21. Your patient is a 78-year-old woman who is complaining of diffuse abdominal pain, nausea, and vomiting. Physical examination reveals abdominal distention and absent bowel sounds. You should suspect she has which of the following conditions?
a. bowel obstruction
b. aortic aneurysm
c. esophageal varices
d. gastrointestinal bleeding

22. Which of the following is NOT an atypical sign and symptom of myocardial infarction that is commonly seen in elderly patients?
a. confusion and fatigue
b. syncope
c. tearing chest pain
d. neck pain

23. Which breathing pattern is characteristic of diabetic ketoacidosis or other types of metabolic acidosis?
a. ataxic breathing
b. Biot's breathing
c. Cheyne-Stokes breathing
d. Kussmaul breathing

24. Your patient is a 70-year-old male. He complains of chest pain that began while he was raking leaves. You perform an initial assessment and a focused history and physical examination and administer oxygen and nitroglycerin. The patient then states that he feels much better. From what is he most likely suffering?
a. stable angina
b. unstable angina
c. myocardial infarction
d. cardiac arrest

25. A 25-year-old female complains of diffuse lower-abdominal pain, vaginal discharge, and low-grade fever. Which of the following conditions best describes the patient's presentation?
a. pelvic inflammatory disease
b. ectopic pregnancy
c. kidney infection
d. ovarian cyst

26. Why are vital sign changes not a good early indicator of shock in a young healthy adult?
a. Patients often display false-positive vital sign readings during shock.
b. The vital signs are often too low to be measured accurately during shock.
c. The body attempts to compensate by maintaining normal vital signs.
d. Signs and symptoms of shock are based on neurological findings only.

27. During an emergency delivery, the newborn's head presents in the canal. After suctioning, how can you assist with the delivery of the anterior shoulder?
a. Gently pull on the infant's head.
b. Gently guide the infant's head upward.
c. Gently guide the infant's head downward.
d. Rotate the infant's head to the transverse position.

28. The physiological cause of the anxiety and restlessness that make up the classic early signs of shock are a direct result of which of the following phenomena?
   a. the release of catecholamines
   b. the decrease in cardiac output
   c. the rise in blood pressure
   d. the constriction of arterioles

Answer questions 29–31 based on the following information.

You arrive to find a 65-year-old male in acute respiratory distress. You hear wheezes from across the room, and you note extreme accessory muscle use. The patient has assumed a tripod position and is breathing through pursed lips. Your physical exam reveals a barrel chest and stained fingernails. Vital signs are blood pressure 160/90 mmHg, pulse 100 BPM, strong and irregular with atrial fibrillation on the cardiac monitor; and respiratory rate 40 breaths per minute with shallow and labored breathing. Auscultation of the chest reveals wheezes and diminished lung sounds throughout all fields.

29. From what is this patient most likely suffering?
   a. chronic bronchitis
   b. anaphylaxis
   c. asthma
   d. emphysema

30. Which of the following medications would NOT be used to treat this patient's condition?
   a. methylprednisolone
   b. albuterol
   c. meperidine
   d. metaproterenol

31. Why is this patient breathing through pursed lips?
   a. to provide positive pressure to inflate the alveoli
   b. to minimize mouth movement during ventilation
   c. to try to retain carbon dioxide in the lung fields
   d. to blow off carbon dioxide to increase blood pH

32. Under what circumstance could the pulse oximetry reading show a falsely elevated reading in a patient?
   a. when the patient is exposed to radioactivity
   b. when the patient is exposed to carbon monoxide
   c. when the patient is exposed to pyrexins
   d. when the patient is exposed to carbon tetrachloride

33. Which technique should you use to open the airway of a trauma patient?
   a. the head-tilt/chin-lift
   b. the jaw thrust
   c. the head-tilt/neck-lift
   d. the sniffing position

34. By what is bronchiolitis caused?
   a. either a bacterial infection or allergy
   b. mycobacterium tuberculosis
   c. respiratory syncytial virus
   d. exacerbation of asthma

Answer questions 35–37 based on the following information.

Your patient is a 30-year-old female who is complaining of a generalized rash and dyspnea after eating shellfish. The patient has small, itchy, red welts all over her body and says her tongue feels like it is swollen. She complains of difficulty moving air in and catching a full breath. This patient's vital signs show a blood pressure of 110/60 mmHg, a pulse of 100 BPM strong and regular, and a respiratory rate of 36 breaths per minute. Her breathing is somewhat shallow and labored.

35. This patient is exhibiting the signs and symptoms of which of the following?
   a. allergic reaction
   b. partial airway obstruction
   c. anaphylactic shock
   d. epiglottitis or croup

36. Medications used to treat this patient may include which of the following?
   a. isoproterenol
   b. haloperidol
   c. hydroxyzine
   d. dopamine

37. This patient needs close monitoring because she could progress into which of the following conditions?
   a. bradycardia
   b. pulmonary edema
   c. anaphylactic shock
   d. respiratory distress

38. After placing an endotracheal tube, you note that breath sounds are much stronger on the right side of the chest than on the left. What does this suggest?
   a. The ET tube has been inserted into the right mainstem bronchus.
   b. The patient has developed a pneumothorax on the right side.
   c. The ET tube has not been inserted far enough into the trachea.
   d. The patient probably has aspirated vomitus into the trachea.

39. You have just delivered a baby girl. Evaluation reveals that the infant cries loudly and has a heart rate of 140. Her body is pink, but the extremities are blue. She is actively moving all extremities. Her Apgar score is which of the following?
   a. 7
   b. 8
   c. 9
   d. 10

40. Causes of third-trimester bleeding include which of the following?
   a. ectopic pregnancy, preeclampsia, uterine rupture
   b. eclampsia, spontaneous abortion, placenta previa
   c. ectopic pregnancy, uterine rupture, pelvic inflammatory disease
   d. abruptio placentae, placenta previa, uterine rupture

41. An assessment finding of pulsus paradoxus is associated with which of the following?
   a. emphysema
   b. congestive heart disease
   c. COPD
   d. myocardial infarction

42. The term *tracheal tugging* refers to which of the following?
   a. the use of accessory muscles during respiration
   b. retraction of intercostal muscles during inspiration
   c. cyanosis and nasal flaring with exhalation
   d. retraction of neck tissues during respiration

43. Your patient is a 66-year-old man who is extremely thin but has a noticeably distorted barrel-shaped chest. He reports a history of dyspnea that has recently gotten worse. You note that he purses his lips when breathing, but hypoxia is not apparent. In addition to monitoring vital signs, breath sounds, obtaining an ECG, starting an IV, and transporting the patient, what other treatments should you give to this patient?
 a. Administer high-flow oxygen via BVM ventilation.
 b. Administer low-flow oxygen and a bronchodilator.
 c. Administer oxygen via nonrebreather mask and furosemide.
 d. Orally intubate the patient and assist ventilations.

44. A 28-year-old woman is complaining of a sudden onset of severe abdominal pain that radiates to her shoulder. Her vital signs are BP 88/60 mmHg, P 110 BPM, and RR 20 breaths per minute. Her skin is cool, pale, and clammy. She states that her last normal menstrual period was 6 to 8 weeks ago. Which of the following conditions best describes the patient presentation?
 a. uterine rupture
 b. ectopic pregnancy
 c. abruptio placentae
 d. perforated uterus

45. What respiratory pattern is characteristic of Kussmaul respiration?
 a. increase in both rate and depth
 b. increase in respiratory rate only
 c. decrease in both rate and depth
 d. decrease in respiratory rate only

46. Which of the following factors increases the amount of energy necessary for the patient to expend for respiration?
 a. loss of pulmonary surfactant
 b. decrease in airway resistance
 c. increase in pulmonary compliance
 d. decrease in body temperature

Answer questions 47–51 based on the following information.

Your patient is a 29-year-old female complaining of the sudden onset of severe shortness of breath and chest pain. She indicates that she is recovering from surgery to her left femur after an automobile crash.

47. From what is this patient most likely suffering?
 a. medication reaction
 b. myocardial infarction
 c. pneumothorax
 d. pulmonary embolism

48. You would expect to find which of the following in this patient?
 a. tracheal deviation
 b. tachycardia
 c. pulses paradoxes
 d. bradypnea

49. This patient's physiological problems are most likely due to what cardiac problem?
 a. right side of the heart pumping against increased resistance
 b. left side of the heart pumping against decreased resistance
 c. right side of the heart pumping against decreased resistance
 d. left side of the heart pumping against increased resistance

50. Proper management of this patient includes which of the following?
   a. IV fluid boluses
   b. low-flow oxygen
   c. administration of bronchodilators
   d. transport in position that places the extremities lower than the heart

51. Which of the following conditions is a common cause of this patient's problem?
   a. placement of a central line
   b. ruptured cerebral aneurism
   c. myocardial tissue damage
   d. anticoagulant drug use

52. Which of the following combinations are the only two situations in which a prehospital provider should place a gloved hand into the vagina?
   a. shoulder dystocia and prolapsed cord
   b. prolapsed cord and a trapped breech presentation
   c. placental abruption and breech presentation
   d. breech presentation and postpartum hemorrhage

53. A patient suspected of showing early signs of shock should usually be placed supine with the patient's feet elevated. When is this position contraindicated?
   a. when a head injury is suspected
   b. if shock is due to hypovolemia
   c. if you suspect respiratory alkalosis
   d. if respirations are inadequate

54. Which statement about deflation of the PASG/MAST in the field setting is correct?
   a. Deflation should be accomplished rapidly in the field.
   b. Deflate the legs first and the abdominal compartment second.
   c. Deflate the garment if the patient begins to experience dyspnea.
   d. Deflation should not be attempted in the field without medical direction.

55. Which of the following statements is true regarding a single limb presentation during an emergency delivery?
   a. Grasp the presenting part of the baby and gently rotate it so the baby will deliver.
   b. This is a nondeliverable presentation and requires immediate transport to an appropriate receiving facility.
   c. Assist the mother in delivering the baby by applying gentle traction to the limb.
   d. Apply firm pressure to the presenting part to delay birth until the patient is transferred to the emergency department staff.

56. How should you position a patient with a suspected stroke and no other pertinent history?
   a. supine with the head raised 15°
   b. in the left-lateral recumbent position
   c. supine with the feet raised 15°
   d. in the right-lateral recumbent position

57. Treatment of an impaled object includes all EXCEPT which one of the following?
   a. controlling bleeding with sterile dressings
   b. providing high-flow supplemental oxygen
   c. removing the object and covering the wound with an occlusive dressing
   d. stabilizing the object with bulky dressings

58. The T wave on an ECG tracing represents which of the following events?
   a. repolarization of the ventricles
   b. depolarization of the atria
   c. depolarization of the ventricles
   d. repolarization of the atria

59. You are analyzing a patient's heart rate on an ECG strip. You note that there are 13 complexes within one 6-second interval. You would record the heart rate as which of the following?
   a. 6
   b. 13
   c. 78
   d. 130

60. Normal atrial depolarization is seen on the Lead II ECG strip as which of the following waveforms?
   a. negative rounded P wave
   b. positive rounded P wave
   c. flattened P wave
   d. biphasic P wave

61. Which of the following is an abnormal finding on an ECG strip?
   a. P-R interval of 0.16 sec
   b. P-R interval of 0.10 sec
   c. QRS complex of 0.10 sec
   d. QRS complex of 0.08 sec

62. An EMS crew attempts to resuscitate a 50-year-old male in cardiac arrest and is not successful. The family sues the EMS organization for negligence. The crew will need to prove that its actions during the resuscitation were
   a. extraordinary and heroic.
   b. not within their duty to act.
   c. in excess of the standards set forth by the American Heart Association.
   d. similar to the actions a reasonably prudent person would do under similar circumstances.

63. How does the Valsalva maneuver improve a too-rapid heartbeat?
   a. It forces the patient to slow down his or her respirations.
   b. It stimulates the vagus nerve to slow the heart rate.
   c. It inhibits the release of acetylcholine, slowing the heart.
   d. It stimulates the carotid artery, slowing blood return.

64. Which dysrhythmia may be a sign of digitalis toxicity?
   a. atrial fibrillation with a ventricular rate of less than 60
   b. premature junctional contractions leading to tachycardia
   c. acute onset paroxysmal supraventricular tachycardia
   d. atrial flutter with a ventricular rate greater than 120

65. Your patient is a stable 67-year-old man who has a pulse and whose ECG strip shows ventricular tachycardia. What should you do after administering oxygen and placing an IV line?
   a. Administer 6 mg of adenosine via rapid IV push.
   b. Administer 2.5–5.0 mg of verapamil via IV.
   c. Sedate and perform synchronized cardioversion.
   d. Administer 1.0–1.5 mg/kg lidocaine via IV.

66. Which of the following is a risk factor for the formation of atherosclerosis?
   a. alcoholism
   b. excessive exercise
   c. diabetes mellitus
   d. cancer

67. Components of an incident command system include all EXCEPT which one of the following?
 a. triage
 b. finance
 c. logistics
 d. command

68. Why are patients who present with pulmonary edema usually assumed to have had a myocardial infarction?
 a. AMI is often the underlying cause of right heart failure.
 b. AMI is frequently a common cause of left ventricle failure.
 c. AMI decreases the oxygen-carrying capacity of the blood.
 d. AMI can result in the formation of a pulmonary embolism.

69. What is the primary goal of management for a patient with left ventricle failure and pulmonary edema?
 a. to decrease cardiac output
 b. to initiate thrombolytic therapy
 c. to decrease venous return
 d. to prevent serious dysrhythmias

70. Your patient is a 68-year-old male with a history of two prior AMIs. Your assessment findings include a pulse rate of 124 BPM, peripheral edema, and jugular vein distention. The patient denies any chest pain or breathing difficulty. What condition should you suspect?
 a. left ventricular failure
 b. right ventricular failure
 c. pulmonary embolism
 d. myocardial infarction

71. Your patient is an 82-year-old female with a suspected MI. While en route to the hospital, you note that her systolic blood pressure, which had been stable, has started to drop, and she is becoming confused. At the same time, her heart rhythm converts to sinus tachycardia. What should you suspect is happening?
 a. She is developing cardiogenic shock.
 b. She is going into sudden cardiac arrest.
 c. Pulmonary edema is causing heart failure.
 d. She has thrown a pulmonary embolus.

72. Which of the following are signs and symptoms of acute pulmonary embolism?
 a. rapid labored breathing and tachycardia
 b. slow labored breathing and cyanosis
 c. acute abdominal pain and anxiety
 d. pallor, chest pain, and tachycardia

73. Your patient is a 67-year-old female who complains of increasing leg pain and tenderness. The skin over the affected area is warm and red, and Homan's sign is positive. Vital signs are unremarkable. How should you treat this patient?
 a. Massage the affected area to relieve the pain and restore circulation.
 b. Elevate the leg and transport the patient for further evaluation.
 c. Give IV fluid boluses to treat the signs and symptoms of shock.
 d. Have the patient walk to the ambulance to promote blood flow.

74. In general, the court deems an emancipated minor to be one who is which of the following?
   1. married
   2. economically independent
   3. maintains a separate home
   4. in the military
   a. 1, 2
   b. 1, 4
   c. 2, 3, 4
   d. 1, 2, 3, 4

75. What is the energy setting for defibrillation in an adult cardiac arrest patient using a monophasic defibrillator?
   a. 100 joules
   b. 200 joules
   c. 300 joules
   d. 360 joules

76. Carotid sinus massage is used for patients with which dysrhythmia?
   a. nonperfusing ventricular tachycardia
   b. refractory ventricular fibrillation
   c. paroxysmal supraventricular tachycardia
   d. second-degree AV block (Mobitz II)

77. External cardiac pacing is used for which of the following rhythms?
   a. ventricular fibrillation
   b. symptomatic bradycardia
   c. PVCs occurring from irritability
   d. PVCs occurring as escape beats

78. What is the usual dosage and route of administration of diazepam given before synchronized cardioversion?
   a. 2–5 mg given intramuscularly
   b. 5–10 mg directly into the vein
   c. 5–15 mg by slow IV push
   d. 10–15 mg administered rectally

79. Which drug is used in management of congestive heart failure?
   a. dobutamine
   b. isoproterenol
   c. bretylium
   d. verapamil

80. Which heart sounds are normal findings on auscultation?
   a. S1 and S2
   b. S2 and S3
   c. S3 and S4
   d. S2 and S4

81. Which set of vital signs is suggestive of left ventricular heart failure with pulmonary edema?
   a. blood pressure elevated, pulse slow and irregular, respirations slow and labored
   b. blood pressure diminished, pulse slow and irregular, respirations rapid but easy
   c. blood pressure diminished, pulse fast and regular, respirations rapid and labored
   d. blood pressure elevated, pulse fast and irregular, respirations rapid and labored

Answer questions 82–87 based on the following information.

You respond for a 44-year-old male diabetic who is complaining of a general feeling of weakness. During your questioning, you learn that he has been "constantly thirsty and hungry." His breath has a fruity odor, and his level of consciousness appears to be diminishing.

82. From which diabetic emergency is this patient most likely suffering?
   a. diabetic ketoacidosis
   b. diabetes mellitus
   c. hypoglycemia
   d. hyperosmolar hyperglycemic nonketotic coma (HHNK)

83. Which vital signs would you expect from this patient?
  a. cool, clammy skin; bradycardia; increased respirations
  b. warm, dry skin; tachycardia; increased respirations
  c. warm, dry skin; bradycardia; decreased respirations
  d. cool, clammy skin; tachycardia; decreased respirations

84. This patient's symptoms are most likely due to which condition?
  a. high levels of insulin
  b. low levels of insulin
  c. low levels of glucose
  d. dehydration

85. Which of the following statements is the most accurate with regard to this patient?
  a. He has not eaten in a while, resulting in hypoglycemia.
  b. He has taken too much insulin, resulting in hyperglycemia.
  c. He has not taken his correct dose of insulin or is ill.
  d. He has taken his insulin but did not regulate his fluid intake.

86. During transport, this patient slips into unconsciousness, and his breathing becomes very deep and rapid. What is this pattern called?
  a. Kussmaul breathing
  b. HHNK respirations
  c. Cheyne-Stokes respirations
  d. Christianson's respirations

87. What does appropriate treatment for this patient include?
  a. IV of D5W or lactated Ringer's solution, oxygen, and IM glucagon
  b. blood glucose test, IV normal saline, and a fluid bolus
  c. blood glucose test, 25 gm of dextrose 50%, and limited fluids
  d. hyperventilation, limited fluids, and sodium bicarbonate

88. Your patient suffers a head trauma that results in a transient loss of consciousness followed by a complete return of function. What is the term for this condition?
  a. cerebral contusion
  b. epidural hematoma
  c. contrecoup injury
  d. cerebral concussion

89. What is the proper procedure for aligning a fractured long bone?
  a. Stabilize the entire limb in the position in which it is found, and then immobilize.
  b. Immobilize the limb with all the joints in the position of function.
  c. Immobilize the distal portion of the limb, and then move the proximal portion.
  d. Stabilize the proximal portion, and then bring the distal portion into alignment.

90. When would you bandage and splint limb injuries on scene?
  a. if the patient does not need rapid transport
  b. if the transport time will be longer than one hour
  c. after treating any life-threatening injuries first
  d. if the fracture has neurovascular compromise

91. What should you do if your examination of a limb suggests that it is fractured?
  a. Apply traction to align the ends of long bones and position the joints.
  b. Treat it as if a fracture exists and immobilize it to prevent further injury.
  c. Check the proximal pulse, motor, and sensation, and adjust the position.
  d. Transport the patient as quickly as possible to preserve function of the limb.

92. Which type of wound would most likely require a tourniquet?
  a. amputation of the hand at the forearm
  b. bilateral open fractures of the femurs
  c. below-the-knee amputation by a machine
  d. tearing injury of the upper arm

93. What is the primary reason that diazepam is given to a seizure patient?
  a. to help relieve any anxiety that may be caused from having a seizure
  b. to suppress the spread of electrical activity in the brain and relax muscles
  c. to prevent hypoglycemia by allowing the brain to effectively use insulin
  d. to help increase the blood pressure by lowering the seizure threshold

94. What is the correct dosage and route of administration of epinephrine for a patient in anaphylaxis?
  a. 0.3–0.5 mg epinephrine 1:10,000, administered subcutaneously
  b. 0.1–0.3 mg epinephrine 1:10,000, administered intravenously
  c. 0.3–0.5 mg epinephrine 1:1,000, administered subcutaneously
  d. 0.1–0.3 mg epinephrine 1:1,000, administered intravenously

95. What is the role of beta-agonists, like albuterol, in the treatment of anaphylaxis?
  a. to relieve anxiety
  b. to prevent shock
  c. to raise blood pressure
  d. to reverse bronchospasm

96. During a multicasualty incident, a conscious patient presents with a fractured femur, a palpable radial pulse, and a respiratory rate of 24/min. According to START, this patient would be placed into what triage category?
  a. minor/green
  b. delayed/yellow
  c. immediate/red
  d. deceased/black

97. What do the symptoms of acetaminophen overdose include?
  a. nausea, vomiting, malaise, diaphoresis, and right upper-quadrant pain
  b. nausea, vomiting, confusion, lethargy, seizures, and dysrhythmias
  c. altered mental status, hypotension, slurred speech, and bradycardia
  d. nausea, dilated pupils, rambling speech, lethargy, headache, and dizziness

98. Prehospital administration of sodium bicarbonate may be ordered for a patient who has overdosed on which of the following drugs?
  a. acetaminophen
  b. benzodiazepines
  c. narcotics
  d. antidepressants

99. Your patient is a 19-year-old female who has been stung by a stingray while swimming. What should you do after ensuring airway breathing and circulation are intact?
- **a.** Apply a tight constricting band between the wound and the heart.
- **b.** Apply heat or warm water to reduce pain and detoxify the poison.
- **c.** Use an icepack wrapped in a towel to relieve pain and swelling.
- **d.** Administer morphine sulfate IM or IV titrated to relieve pain.

100. Which drug can cause users to behave violently and aggressively?
- **a.** amitriptyline
- **b.** phenobarbital
- **c.** PCP
- **d.** LSD

101. Which of the following patients shows signs and symptoms of heat exhaustion?
- **a.** male, age 34: severe muscle cramps in legs and abdomen, fatigue, and dizziness
- **b.** female, age 45: rapid, shallow respirations; weak pulse; cool, clammy skin; dizziness
- **c.** male, age 42: deep respirations; rapid, strong pulse; dry, hot skin; loss of consciousness
- **d.** female, age 70: shallow respirations; weak, rapid pulse; dilated pupils; seizures

102. Which of the following statements about care of a prolonged water submersion victim is correct?
- **a.** The Heimlich maneuver should be used to clear the airway.
- **b.** Ventilation should not be provided until the patient is clear of the water.
- **c.** The patient should be admitted to the hospital for observation.
- **d.** Drowning victims seldom experience head or neck injury.

103. You are interviewing a 43-year-old woman with a long history of schizophrenia. She appears to try to cooperate, but there are long periods of silence in your conversation while she listens to her "voices." How should you respond during her silence?
- **a.** Repeat your last question.
- **b.** Restate her last response.
- **c.** Remain quietly attentive.
- **d.** Tell an interesting story.

104. A patient with bipolar disorder usually suffers from which of the following?
- **a.** frequent hallucinations
- **b.** delusional behavior
- **c.** wide mood swings
- **d.** psychotic thoughts

Answer questions 105–107 based on the following information.

You respond to a 12-year-old male who is wheezing and having difficulty breathing. The patient has a long history of asthma and states that he used his inhaler but that it did not help much. Upon examination, you discover that the patient is tachycardic and tachypneic with a nonproductive cough.

105. What is the primary goal in treating this patient?
- **a.** correct hypoxia, reverse bronchospasms, and decrease inflammation
- **b.** decrease respiratory drive, decrease heart rate, and increase blood pressure
- **c.** increase heart rate, decrease respiratory rate, and correct carbon dioxide levels
- **d.** correct carbon dioxide levels, decrease inflammation, and increase heart rate

106. All of these triggers may have produced the patient's condition EXCEPT which one of the following?
a. warm air
b. allergens
c. exercise
d. medications

107. Treatment for this patient includes which of the following medications?
a. midazolam, epinephrine, and diazepam
b. albuterol, aminophylline, and atropine
c. albuterol, ipratropium, and steroids
d. terbutaline, steroids, and verapamil

108. Diazapam and lorazepam are examples of which of the following?
a. antipsychotics
b. phenothiazines
c. tricyclic antidepressants
d. benzodiazepines

109. A five-year-old male has multiple injuries in various stages of healing, including raccoon eyes and a newly suspected broken leg. On questioning, his mother states that he fell out of his bunk bed. However, his sister, age nine, says, "Daddy beat him." The mother insists that her husband will take the child to the hospital when he gets home from work. How should you proceed?
a. Document your findings, convince the mother that transport to the hospital is necessary, and report your suspicions of child abuse.
b. Make sure his condition is stable, grant the mother's request for delayed transport, and follow up that evening to confirm that treatment was sought.
c. Confront the mother with your suspicions, transport the child immediately, and call the police.
d. Remove both children from the home immediately and transport both of them to the hospital for a complete evaluation.

110. A physician at the scene of an incident instructs you to provide care for a patient that you know to be inappropriate given the patient's present condition. Your best course of action will be to
a. Contact the medical control physician and ask him to speak with the on-scene physician.
b. Inform the on-scene physician that you disagree with his instructions and ask him to perform the procedures himself.
c. Politely inform the physician that his instructions are inappropriate and ask him to leave the room.
d. Ignore the on-scene physician's order, load the patient in the ambulance as quickly as possible, and transport rapidly to the hospital.

Answer questions 111–114 based on the following information.

You respond to the residence of a four-year-old male who was found in his backyard, head down in a five-gallon bucket of water. The child, according to the mother, was in the water for approximately four minutes. The child is cyanotic, pulseless, and apneic. The ECG shows his heart is in asystole. The child weighs approximately 40 pounds.

111. Which of the following would be the most reliable method for determining the proper medication dosing for this pediatric patient?
a. Give no more than $\frac{1}{2}$ the adult dose for all medications.
b. Give $\frac{1}{3}$ the adult dose for all medications except atropine.
c. Use the Broselow tape or another length-weight measuring system.
d. Estimate the patient's kilogram weight by dividing by 2.2.

112. You unsuccessfully have tried three times to establish a peripheral IV in this patient. Which of the following is the most preferred route to administer medications if a peripheral IV is not available?
a. endotracheal tube
b. external jugular access
c. intraosseous access
d. rectal access

113. After endotracheal intubation of this patient, which of the following steps should be done first?
a. Confirm the ETT placement.
b. Inflate the cuff to prevent air leakage.
c. Dilute all ETT medication to 10 mL.
d. Tape the tube to the patient's maxilla.

114. After the first round of ACLS drugs, the patient converts to a sinus bradycardia at a rate of 40 beats per minute. What is the drug of choice for managing this patient's bradycardia?
a. epinephrine
b. atropine
c. isoproterenol
d. dobutamine

115. Knee injuries and hip dislocations that occur during a motor vehicle crash are often the result of which pathway of energy transfer?
a. down and under
b. down and back
c. up and over
d. up and back

116. A high-velocity bullet passes through the body. Besides the direct damage caused by the bullet, what other related condition could cause harm to the patient?
a. the type of metal used to make the bullet
b. the internal opening created by cavitation
c. the gunpowder residue
d. the length of the bullet

117. An injury to the brain opposite the site of a blunt force impact is called which of the following?
a. contralateral
b. concussion
c. contrecoup
d. coup force

118. One way to determine the size of the endotracheal tube to use in a child is to use the following equation: 16 plus the child's age divided by 4. What also might be considered to determine the size of the endotracheal tube?
a. glottic opening
b. pleural space
c. pharynx
d. cricoid cartilage

119. A 17-year-old male complains of a steadily worsening headache several days after being struck in the head during football practice. Which of the following injuries best describes this patient's presentation?
   a. concussion
   b. subdural hematoma
   c. epidural hematoma
   d. subarachnoid bleed

120. When should you examine a woman, who is about to give birth, for crowning?
   a. during a contraction
   b. between contractions
   c. during an internal pelvic exam
   d. only when time permits

121. Your patient is a 32-year-old woman who reports that she is 14 weeks pregnant. She complains of abdominal cramping and vaginal bleeding. How should you proceed?
   a. Perform an internal vaginal exam and treat her for any signs of ectopic pregnancy.
   b. Administer high-flow oxygen, monitor fetal heart tones, and transport immediately.
   c. Treat for signs and symptoms of hypovolemia, provide emotional support, and transport.
   d. Position the patient supine, open an OB kit, and prepare for emergency delivery in the field.

122. What is the cause of the supine hypotensive syndrome in the pregnant patient?
   a. pressure of the uterus on the inferior vena cava
   b. normal volume depletion during pregnancy
   c. the occurrence of abruptio placentae
   d. abnormal fetal presentation or positioning

123. Which of the following is a differential sign or symptom of spinal shock associated with trauma?
   a. an elevated heart rate
   b. decreasing blood pressure
   c. anxiety or sense of doom
   d. warm, dry skin distal to the injury site

124. During a normal delivery, you would tell the mother to stop pushing when
   a. crowning begins.
   b. the head is delivered.
   c. delivery of the infant is complete.
   d. the placenta is delivered.

125. What is the appropriate treatment for a prolapsed cord?
   a. Attempt to push the cord back into the vagina and deliver the infant normally.
   b. Place two fingers on either side of the baby's nose and mouth and lift the head until it is delivered.
   c. Place two fingers to raise the presenting part of the fetus off the cord, place the mother in knee-chest position, administer oxygen, and transport.
   d. Assist and support the mother for a normal vaginal delivery.

126. Immediately after delivery, how should you position the neonate?
a. higher than the mother's vagina, with the head slightly elevated
b. at the level of the mother's vagina, with the head slightly lower than the body
c. lower than the mother's vagina, with the head at the same level as the body
d. at the level of the mother's vagina, with the head slightly elevated

127. A patient who complains of a sudden and painless complete loss of vision in one eye is most likely suffering from which of the following?
a. acute retinal artery occlusion
b. retinal detachment
c. conjunctival hemorrhage
d. hyphema

128. What is the first step in the resuscitation of a distressed neonate?
a. Ventilate with 100% oxygen for 15–30 seconds.
b. Administer naloxone.
c. Evaluate breath sounds.
d. Initiate chest compressions.

129. Which of the following statements about supplying supplemental oxygen to a neonate is incorrect?
a. Do not withhold oxygen from a neonate in the prehospital setting.
b. Oxygen toxicity in the prehospital setting is a serious concern.
c. Administer supplemental oxygen by blowing it across the neonate's face.
d. Oxygen should be warmed if possible prior to administration.

130. How much intravenous fluid should you administer to a distressed neonate who weighs 2 kg?
a. 10 mL
b. 20 mL
c. 30 mL
d. 40 mL

131. A patient was hit several times in the left chest with the large end of a pool cue. The patient is in severe respiratory distress with tachycardia and tachypnea. Crepitus can be felt in multiple locations over the left anterior fourth, fifth, sixth, and seventh rib area. Lung sounds are clear and equal, but diminished. Which of the following conditions best describes the patient's presentation?
a. flail chest
b. tension pneumothorax
c. pericardial tamponade
d. pulmonary contusion

132. A patient is found lying supine on the floor with a stab wound to her right anterior chest just below the breast. The patient is having difficulty breathing and has cool and clammy skin. No jugular venous distention (JVD) is noted. Breath sounds are absent over the right side. This patient most likely is experiencing which of the following?
a. pneumothorax
b. pericardial tamponade
c. tension pneumothorax
d. hemothorax

Answer questions 133–137 based on the following information.

You respond to reports of a bus collision. Upon arrival, it appears that you have approximately 35 patients.

133. What is your first priority?
  a. Set up the triage close to the treatment and transport areas.
  b. Establish the morgue area away from the view of the patients.
  c. Begin rapid treatment of the most seriously injured patients.
  d. Separate the walking wounded from the more severely injured.

134. The first parameter to assess when using the START algorithm should be which of the following?
  a. pulse
  b. breathing/airway
  c. respiratory rate
  d. level of consciousness

135. A male patient is found to have a respiratory rate of 38. This would place him in which of the following categories?
  a. delayed
  b. immediate
  c. expectant/deceased
  d. minor

136. Another male patient is found to have a respiratory rate of 28 breaths per minute and a radial pulse of 84 BPM. He is confused about the incident. This patient would be placed in which of the following categories?
  a. delayed
  b. immediate
  c. expectant
  d. minor

137. A female patient is found to have no spontaneous respirations. What should you do next?
  a. Use a bag-valve mask and ventilate with 100% oxygen.
  b. Assess for a pulse.
  c. Reposition the airway and check her again for respirations.
  d. Start CPR and call for immediate removal to the treatment area.

138. What is the legal term for an intentional deviation from the accepted standard of care that results in harm to a patient?
  a. negligence
  b. liability
  c. res ipsa loquitur
  d. abandonment

139. A wrestler feels his shoulder "pop" when his opponent twists his arm during a hold. There is immediate pain and loss of range of motion in the shoulder. What is the patient's likely injury?
  a. subluxation
  b. muscle strain
  c. torn ligament
  d. torn rotator cuff

140. Which of the following statements is INCORRECT regarding the care of patients who are contaminated by hazardous material?
  a. Trained personnel should immediately remove nonambulatory patients from the hot zone.
  b. Decontamination activities should be carried out while the patient is in the warm zone.
  c. Intravenous therapy and invasive procedures should begin only under specific physician direction.
  d. An initial assessment should be done while the patient is located within the hot zone.

141. Using the START method at a multiple-casualty accident scene, you encounter a patient who is making no spontaneous respiratory effort despite attempts at repositioning. What should you do next?
   a. Tag the patient as expectant/deceased and move on.
   b. Request medical backup from the treatment area.
   c. Begin mouth to mask or bag-valve mask ventilation.
   d. Move the patient to the care area and intubate.

142. A 72-year-old man trips and falls while walking to his bathroom. Physical findings include a lateral rotation of the left foot and knee. The patient has tenderness and a protrusion in the left groin area. You suspect which of the following?
   a. distal femur fracture
   b. anterior dislocation of the hip
   c. ischial tuberosity fracture
   d. posterior dislocation of the hip

143. When is use of *reasonable* force or use of restraints permissible for a patient?
   a. The patient is alert and cooperative, but anxious.
   b. The patient has an altered level of conscious and is demonstrating violent/hostile behavior toward themselves or others.
   c. It is never appropriate to use any force on a patient.
   d. This is at the discretion of the paramedic or the crew's officer.

144. Primary injuries from a blast include which of the following?
   a. extremity fractures
   b. organ lacerations
   c. impaled objects
   d. lung injuries

145. What is the rhythm in Figure 5.2?
   a. first-degree AV block
   b. sinus arrest
   c. third-degree AV block
   d. second-degree AV block Mobitz type II

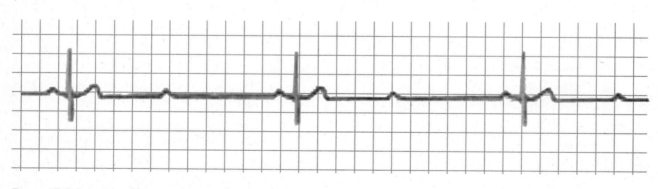

Figure 5.2 Reprinted by permission from WSUPharmacy2015 (2012).

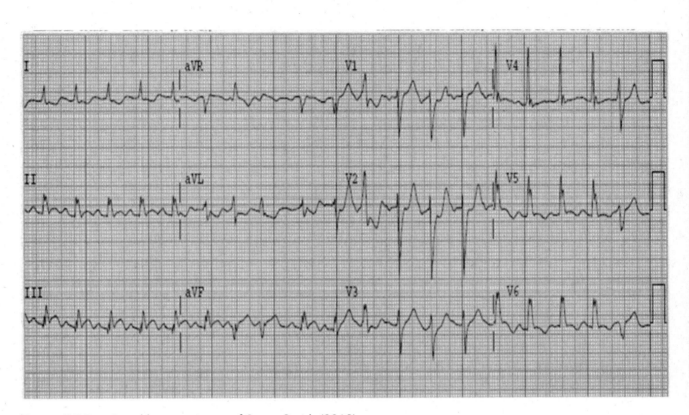

Figure 5.3 Reprinted by permisson of Steve Smith (2010).

146. What is the location of the infarct in the 12-lead ECG in Figure 5.3?
　　a. inferior wall MI with left ventricular hypertrophy
　　b. left bundle branch block with an undetermined MI
　　c. septal wall MI
　　d. right bundle branch block with inferior wall MI

147. What is the rhythm in Figure 5.4?
　　a. sinus tachycardia
　　b. ventricular tachycardia
　　c. sinus arrhythmia
　　d. supraventricular tachycardia

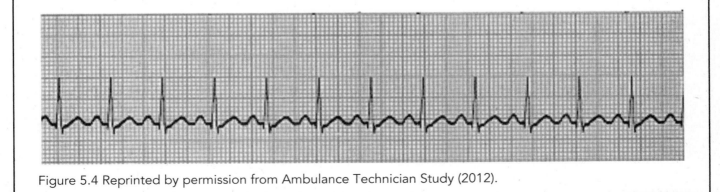

Figure 5.4 Reprinted by permission from Ambulance Technician Study (2012).

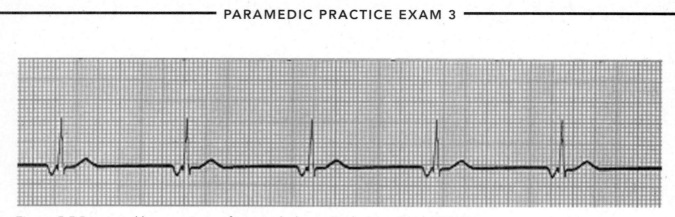

Figure 5.5 Reprinted by permission from Ambulance Technician Study (2012).

148. What is the rhythm in Figure 5.5?
   a. sinus rhythm with a wandering pacemaker
   b. sinus bradycardia
   c. normal sinus rhythm
   d. junctional rhythm

149. Which of the following is a contraindication to the administration of succinylcholine?
   a. hypercalcemia
   b. hyperkalemia
   c. hyperglycemia
   d. hypercoaguable state

150. On which of the following patients would you want to consider prolonging the expiratory phase as you adjust the I:E ratio on your ventilator?
   a. a patient with reactive airway disease
   b. a patient with a head injury
   c. a newborn with difficulty breathing
   d. a patient with a high spinal cord injury

Answers

1. b. This choice lists the organs that can be palpated in the right upper quadrant (liver, gall bladder, head of the pancreas, part of the duodenum, and part of the colon).

2. a. Stable angina is caused by a temporary low-flow state in the coronary arteries that does not lead to cell injury or death (infarction). During hypoperfusion, lactic acid and excessive carbon dioxide are not carried away, causing irritation and pain.

3. b. Due to the low blood pressure, this patient would be classified as unstable. Immediate intervention will be needed to correct this condition. Delivering medications may take too long to administer. Defibrillation may invoke ventricular fibrillation.

4. c. Pulse pressure refers to the difference between the systolic and diastolic blood pressure readings. A narrowing pulse pressure indicates increasing diastolic pressure and decreasing systolic pressure. Perfusion will stop once both pressures come together.

5. b. The patient's heart is not pumping efficiently, possibly due to an MI. This would result in a loss of blood pressure throughout the cardiovascular system, including the pulmonary vessels. The lack of pressure causes plasma to leak into the interstitial space of the lungs, causing the adventitious breath sounds.

6. b. A sudden loss of blood flow to the leg within the arterial bed would account for the sudden change in skin color and temperature.

7. b. This set of vitals, known as Cushing's triad (respiratory rate is irregular or decreased, heart rate decreased, blood pressure increased), is common in closed head injuries.

8. a. A c-spine injury should be assumed until proven otherwise. The patient has full deep respirations at a rate of 24 indicating an open and clear airway. This patient has suffered a head injury and therefore does not require a fluid challenge.

9. d. Choices **a**, **b**, and **c** are all common in closed head injuries; choice **d** (hemopneumothorax) is not.

10. b. A patient with a detached retina will often complain of seeing a dark curtain in front of part of the field of vision.

11. c. Although the patient may be complaining of chest discomfort, administering nitroglycerin would only worsen an already low blood pressure. Even with fluid leaking into the interstitial lung tissue secondary to the low blood pressure in the pulmonary circulation, a diuretic would also carry the same risk of reducing pressure even more. This patient requires a vasoactive medication such as dopamine to increase blood pressure.

12. b. Traumatic asphyxia occurs when a serious rib injury pushes the chest wall inward, resulting in severe hypoventilation and backflow of venous blood. Important signs and symptoms of this include dyspnea, bloodshot eyes, distended neck veins, and a cyanotic upper body.

13. b. The total body surface area is 18%. According to the rule of nines, the head and upper back are each equal to 9% of body surface area.

14. c. This is often the appearance of a third-degree burn, which is painless because of destruction of nerve cells.

15. d. The vital signs listed in choice **d** indicate the presence of shock. An isolated injury of penetrating trauma to the upper arm is not generally life threatening. A 10-mile-per-hour impact to a pedestrian is not generally a significant MOI. Burns to the entire chest cover a body surface area of approximately 9%; this would not in itself require rapid transport unless other problems existed.

16. c. Eye opening = 2; verbal response = 2; motor response = 4.

17. d. These are the classic signs and symptoms of appendicitis.

18. b. The abdominal aorta is located in the retroperitoneal space. A sudden loss of pressure due to an aortic aneurysm will result in loss of perfusion below the site of injury.

19. a. This patient is suffering from second-degree AV block type 1 (Wenckebach), which is an intermittent block at the AV node. There is generally no treatment necessary for stable patients with second-degree AV heart block type I other than oxygen and monitoring.

20. a. Although symptoms of full-blown AIDS include Kaposi's sarcoma and opportunistic infections, initial symptoms of infection with the AIDS virus often consist only of mild fatigue and fever.

21. a. The patient is displaying signs and symptoms of bowel obstruction.

22. c. There are many atypical signs and symptoms of MI in elderly patients; choices **a**, **b**, and **d** list three of them. A tearing sensation in the chest generally indicates a dissecting aneurysm is occurring.

23. d. Kussmaul breathing is characteristic of diabetic ketoacidosis.

24. a. The pain of stable angina is brought on by exertion and relieved by rest, oxygen, and nitroglycerin.

25. a. PID causes lower-abdominal discomfort that is difficult to localize and often has an associated fever. Pain associated with an ectopic pregnancy is more localized, as is the pain associated with solid organ involvement.

26. c. The body's physiological mechanisms compensate for the insult that causes shock. Therefore, although changes in vital signs are ominous late signs in patients with poor tissue perfusion, they are unlikely to occur in a young healthy adult who has just entered a state of shock.

27. c. The head will tend to drop down as the shoulders begin to pass through the birth canal. The paramedic can gently guide the head to help with the process.

28. a. The release of catecholamines that results from the initial drop in blood pressure causes the feelings of anxiety and restlessness.

29. d. This patient is exhibiting the classic signs and symptoms of emphysema.

30. c. Meperidine is not indicated for this patient.

31. a. Breathing through pursed lips is a common compensatory mechanism COPD patients use to provide positive end-expiratory pressure (PEEP), which forces more alveoli to inflate.

32. b. Carbon monoxide poisoning can cause a falsely high pulse oximetry reading.

33. b. The jaw thrust is used to open the airway of patients with suspected cervical spine injury. Any trauma patient with questionable or unknown mechanism of injury should be assumed to have a cervical spine injury until it is ruled out.

34. c. The respiratory syncytial virus, which causes only mild upper-respiratory infections in older persons, causes bronchiolitis, a serious respiratory infection, in infants and young children.

35. a. This patient's blood pressure is still compensating for the allergic reaction; therefore, the patient is not in anaphylactic shock.

36. c. Isoproterenol, haloperidol, and dopamine are not indicated for this patient. Hydroxyzine is an antihistamine that can be used to treat the puritis (itchy red welts).

37. c. This patient needs to be monitored for possible anaphylactic shock.

38. a. If breath sounds are stronger on one side than on the other, or absent on one side, this suggests that the tube has been inserted too far and is resting in one bronchus.

39. c. With the exception of the blue extremities, the infant scores a 2 on activity, pulse, grimace, and respirations. Her appearance score is a 1.

40. d. A ruptured ectopic pregnancy usually occurs within the first trimester. Eclampsia and PID are not associated with bleeding.

41. c. Pulsus paradoxus, or a drop in blood pressure with each respiratory cycle, is associated with chronic obstructive pulmonary disease (COPD).

42. d. *Tracheal tugging* refers to retraction of neck tissues during respiratory effort.

43. b. The patient is showing signs and symptoms of emphysema. Administer low-flow oxygen to preserve his hypoxic drive.

44. b. A sudden rupture of an ectopic pregnancy would result in a loss of blood that would place the patient in compensatory shock.

45. a. Kussmaul respiration, which is associated with diabetic ketoacidosis, is characterized by increased rate and depth of respirations.

46. a. Loss of pulmonary surfactant, which can occur in pneumonia and other conditions, increases the tendency of the alveoli to collapse and, thus, increases the work necessary for respiration.

47. d. This patient has symptoms of a pulmonary embolism.

48. b. You would expect to see this patient with tachycardia rather than bradycardia due to the increasing dyspnea and hypoxia resulting from the pulmonary embolism.

49. a. The pulmonary embolism has caused the right side of the heart to have to pump harder against a resistance caused by the partial blockage. This results in the severe shortness of breath and hypoxia.

50. d. This patient should be transported in the position in which it is easiest for her to breathe (i.e., high Fowler's with extremities lower than the heart).

51. a. Ruptured aneurism, myocardial infarction, and anticoagulant drug use are not common causes of pulmonary embolism.

52. b. In both of these cases, relieving pressure off the trapped umbilical cord (prolapsed) or the face and airway passages (trapped breech) may be the life-saving measure.

53. a. The shock position is used only if head injury is not suspected.

54. d. Because the PASG corrects a symptom and not the underlying problem, deflation should be attempted only in the hospital after the underlying hypovolemia is corrected.

55. b. A limb presentation during delivery requires a cesarean section to complete the delivery. Provide high-flow oxygen and care to the mother during transport.

56. a. The patient should be supine with the head elevated to enhance venous return. If congestive heart failure is present, the patient should be positioned at least semi-Fowler's (sitting up at least 45°).

57. c. The object should not be removed from the patient, but stabilized with bulky dressings. The rare exception is if the object or associated bleeding is obstructing the airway.

58. a. The T wave on the ECG reflects the repolarization of the ventricles.

59. d. Calculate the rate by multiplying the number of complexes in a 6-second interval by 10. The heart rate is 130.

60. b. Normal atrial depolarization is represented in Lead II as a positive rounded P wave.

61. b. A normal P-R interval is 0.12–0.20 seconds; a normal QRS complex lasts 0.04–0.12 seconds.

62. d. The "reasonable person" standard sets a minimum guideline for what similarly trained personnel would do under similar circumstances—in this case, a cardiac arrest. As long as the crew could demonstrate that its actions were reasonable and expected to be done by other prehospital-care providers in a similar situation, this would avoid a negligence allegation.

63. b. The Valsalva maneuver (bearing down against a closed glottis) stimulates the vagus nerve, which innervates the heart.

64. a. Atrial fibrillation with a low ventricular rate is suggestive of digitalis toxicity.

65. d. Lidocaine is the first-choice drug for perfusing ventricular tachycardia.

66. c. Risk factors for atherosclerosis include diabetes, advanced age, obesity, lack of exercise, hypertension, and smoking.

67. a. C-FLOP is a mnemonic used to describe the components of an ICS system: command—finance, logistics, operations, planning.

68. b. Myocardial infarction is a common cause of left ventricular failure, which is closely associated with pulmonary edema.

69. c. The primary goal for patients with left ventricular failure and pulmonary edema is to reduce venous return to the heart, or preload, and thus reduce pressure on the pulmonary circulation.

70. b. The patient's history, signs, and symptoms suggest right ventricular failure.

71. a. Signs of cardiogenic shock include a sudden drop in systolic blood pressure and increasing confusion.

72. a. Rapid labored breathing and tachycardia are the most common signs of a pulmonary embolism; onset is usually sudden, and there may or may not be chest pain.

73. b. The clinical picture suggests deep venous thrombosis. The correct action is to elevate the leg and transport the patient for further evaluation. Do not massage the area or allow the patient to walk, since pulmonary emboli may be provoked.

74. d. Each of the answers defines an emancipated minor.

75. d. 2010 AHA guidelines eliminated stacked shocks; all defibrillations are set at 360 joules or the highest energy level in an automated external defibrillator (AED).

76. c. Carotid sinus massage can convert PSVTs by increasing vagal tone and decreasing heart rate.

77. b. External cardiac pacing is used to correct symptomatic bradycardias by directing the heart's electrical system.

78. c. Five to 15 mg by slow IV push is the correct dosage and route when diazepam is used to relax the patient and cause amnesia before cardioversion.

79. a. Dobutamine is used in patients with congestive heart failure to increase stroke volume, and in that way, increase cardiac output.

80. a. S1 and S2 are normal sounds; extra sounds are abnormal findings.

81. d. These vital signs (blood pressure elevated, pulse fast and irregular, respirations rapid and labored) are consistent with left ventricular failure with pulmonary edema.

82. a. These are symptoms of diabetic ketoacidosis.

83. b. Warm, dry skin; tachycardia; and increased respirations are common vitals seen in keto-acidotic patients.

84. b. Ketoacidotic patients have low levels of insulin.

85. c. Most likely, this patient has not taken his insulin or has an infection that upset the glucose-insulin balance.

86. a. Kussmaul breathing is very deep and rapid; it represents the body's attempt to compensate for the metabolic acidosis produced by the ketones and organic acids in the blood.

87. b. The appropriate treatment for this patient would be a blood glucose test, an IV of isotonic crystalloid solution like normal saline or lactated Ringer's, and an initial fluid bolus of 500 mL.

88. d. A concussion is a brief loss of consciousness in response to head trauma.

89. d. Use gentle traction to bring the distal part of the limb into alignment with the proximal part.

90. a. If the patient's condition is such that rapid transport is necessary, you would care for limb injuries while en route, rather than completing a detailed physical exam and bandaging and splinting on scene.

91. b. You cannot harm a patient by immobilizing a limb properly, but you may possibly cause further injury by failing to immobilize a fracture. Always assess the distal pulse before and after splinting.

92. d. Because a tearing wound can tear multiple large blood vessels, bleeding may be particularly difficult to control and a tourniquet may be necessary. Clean amputations often do not require a tourniquet.

93. b. Although diazepam (Valium) does reduce anxiety, it is given to seizure patients to suppress the spread of electrical activity through the brain, as well as to relax the muscles.

94. c. The correct dosage and route of administration (0.3–0.5 mg epinephrine 1:1,000, administered subcutaneously) is given. Always follow local protocols, as some may allow 0.3–0.5 mg of epinephrine 1:10,000 via IV per standing orders or by contacting medical control.

95. d. Beta-agonists, such as albuterol, are most frequently used in the treatment of reactive airway disease (asthma). They are also used to prevent or relieve bronchospasm and laryngeal edema in patients with anaphylaxis. Beta blockers are often used to control hypertension, but beta-agonists are not used to raise blood pressure, making choice **c** incorrect.

96. b. According to START principles, transport of this patient to definitive care can be delayed. He is breathing spontaneously, has a radial pulse, and is conscious. The fractured femur is not factored into the evaluation of transport status.

97. a. These are the most common symptoms of acetaminophen overdose.

98. d. Sodium bicarbonate is sometimes ordered in the field for ingestions of tricyclic antidepressants with cardiac symptoms (wide complex tachycardias).

99. b. Heat will cause the poison to break down and lessen the harm to the patient.

100. c. PCP can cause bizarre delusions as well as violent and uncontrollable behavior.

101. b. Rapid, shallow respirations; weak pulse; cold, clammy skin; and dizziness are signs and symptoms of heat exhaustion. Patient **a** shows signs of heat cramps and patients **c** and **d** show signs and symptoms of heat stroke.

102. c. Due to the chance of post-event pulmonary edema, all prolonged submersion victims should be admitted to the hospital for observation.

103. c. During silences, remain relaxed and attentive and wait to hear what the patient has to say. This will encourage the patient to talk.

104. c. A patient with bipolar disorder (manic-depressive disorder) suffers from wide mood swings from euphoria to debilitating depression.

105. a. The goal with this asthma patient would be to correct hypoxia, reverse bronchospasms, and decrease inflammation.

106. a. Cold air, not warm air, is a common trigger for asthma. Choices **b**, **c**, and **d** are also triggers.

107. c. Albuterol, ipratropium, and/or steroids are commonly used in the treatment of asthma.

108. d. Diazepam (Valium) and lorazepam (Ativan) are benzodiazepines, which have sedative effects and are prescribed for patients who suffer from acute anxiety attacks.

109. a. In cases of suspected child abuse, your responsibility is to ensure that the patient receives necessary care immediately and report your findings.

110. a. The medical control physician should be able to engage with the on-scene physician to discuss the patient's condition, the level of care that will be provided by the EMS personnel, and the transportation destination options.

111. c. Using the Broselow tape or another length-weight measuring system is the most appropriate way to determine proper medication for a pediatric patient.

112. c. Intraosseous is the preferred access route in pediatric patients if intravenous access is not readily available.

113. a. Your first step following placement of the ET tube is to confirm its placement in the trachea. After confirmation of placement, secure the tube with tape or use a commercial device to help prevent dislodging of the tube. Pay especially close attention to these tubes as they are easily displaced, even when secured. Depending on which size tube you use, it may or may not be a cuffed tube. Medication administration will follow after confirmation that the tube is placed and secure.

114. a. Epinephrine is indicated for pediatric bradycardia in this situation.

115. a. During a frontal crash, the down-and-under pathway causes the knees to strike the lower dashboard violently, causing the described injury pattern.

116. b. Cavitation caused by the pressure wave of the bullet's force creates both temporary and permanent openings within the tissues. Tremendous force is transferred from the velocity of the bullet to the tissues, causing damage.

117. c. During significant force to the head, the brain can shift and strike the opposite side of the skull away from the original force. This mechanism can cause a contrecoup injury.

118. d. In addition to the child's age, the size of the endotracheal tube should be based on the size of the cricoid cartilage, which is the narrowest part of a child's airway.

119. b. A subdural bleed occurs when a small vein bleeds into the area below the dura mater. It may take some time before pressure from the bleeding is high enough to cause clinical signs and symptoms.

120. a. Look for crowning, or the appearance of the baby's head at the opening of the vagina, only during a contraction.

121. c. The patient is most likely suffering a miscarriage. Treat her for signs and symptoms of shock due to blood loss, provide emotional support, retain any clumps of tissue she passes, and transport.

122. a. Supine hypotensive syndrome, a normal occurrence during late pregnancy, is caused by the pressure of the pregnant uterus on the inferior vena cava when the patient is supine.

123. d. While the other answers are signs and symptoms of shock, only choice **d** reflects a specific sign that points directly to the underlying cause of hypoperfusion.

124. b. To avoid a precipitous delivery, tell the mother to stop pushing after the head is delivered.

125. c. To treat a prolapsed cord, place two fingers of a gloved hand to raise the presenting part of the fetus off the cord; then, place the mother in Trendelenburg or knee-chest position, administer high-flow oxygen, and transport immediately.

126. b. Position the neonate at the level of the mother's vagina, with the neonate's head slightly lower than the body to facilitate drainage of secretions.

127. b. The retina captures the image that is projected by the lens of the eye. It can spontaneously separate from the inner surface of the eye, causing sudden and painless loss of vision.

128. a. Ventilate with 100% oxygen; then, evaluate the heart rate and initiate chest compressions if necessary.

129. b. Oxygen toxicity occurs only if oxygen is administered for several days; do not withhold oxygen in the prehospital setting.

130. b. Fluid therapy for a neonate consists of 10 mL/kg (20 mL for a 2 kg neonate), administered via syringe over a 5- to 10-minute period.

131. a. Flail chest is very possible in this case, due to the mechanism of injury. The lack of other signs or symptoms such as jugular venous distension or unequal or absent breath sounds minimizes the possibilities of a pneumothorax or tamponade.

132. d. The lack of jugular venous distension in the supine position is very telling; it suggests a large loss of volume from the circulatory system.

133. d. According to the START method, separating the walking wounded from the more severely injured patients is the first step in triaging large numbers of patients.

134. b. Breathing/airway is the first parameter that should be assessed, followed by pulse and mental status.

135. b. The START triage acronym dictates that patients with respiratory rates above 30 be classified as immediate.

136. b. The decreased level of consciousness places the patient in the immediate category. Once he is moved to the treatment area, he may be monitored or transported quickly.

137. c. Reposition the head and examine for spontaneous respirations. If they are immediately present, categorize the patient as immediate. If they are absent, categorize the patient as expectant/deceased and move on to the next patient.

138. a. Negligence refers to an intentional deviation from the accepted standard of care that results in harm to a patient.

139. a. A subluxation of the shoulder is a partial dislocation of the joint, due to injuries sustained by the rotator cuff during a severe twisting force to the joint.

140. d. Only absolutely essential care, such as ABCs and spinal immobilization, should be done in the hot zone.

141. a. If a patient continues to remain apneic following a second attempt to open the airway, the patient is considered unsalvageable.

142. b. The outward rotation of the left extremity along with the deformity in the groin area points to an anterior dislocation injury.

143. b. If the patient is altered and is placing the patient's own safety or others' in harm's way, the EMS provider should use any method within reason to control the patient's actions.

144. d. Tertiary blast injuries are caused by the victim being propelled away from the blast and into objects on the ground. Injuries from this are similar to those sustained from ejection from an automobile. Primary blast injuries result from compression of hollow organs such as the lungs. Secondary blast injuries are caused by flying debris propelled by the force of the blast.

145. d. The rhythm is a second-degree AV block Mobitz type II. Each QRS has a P wave that is nonconducted. In second-degree AV block Mobitz type I, the PR interval lengthens until a QRS complex is dropped. In third-degree there is no correlation between the P waves and the QRS complexes.

146. b. This 12-lead ECG shows a left bundle branch block, which prevents any further interpretation. The R waves in V1–V6 do not indicate left ventricular hypertrophy. Although there may be ST elevation in leads II, III, and AVF, it is not a right bundle branch block. The inferior wall MI cannot be confirmed due to the left bundle branch block.

147. a. The rhythm is sinus tachycardia. The rate is greater than 100 and there are distinct P waves for each QRS. The QRS complexes are less than 0.12 seconds, which eliminates ventricular tachycardia. Sinus arrhythmia has an irregular rhythm. The rate is 120, which is generally too slow to be considered supraventricular tachycardia.

148. d. The rhythm is a junctional rhythm. The rate is less than 60 and the P waves are inverted. The P-R interval is constant, so there is no wandering pacemaker. The inverted P waves are not consistent with sinus bradycardia. It cannot be normal sinus rhythm due to the bradycardic rate.

149. b. Hyperkalemia is a contraindication to the administration of succinylcholine. Succinylcholine can cause a release of potassium, further amplifying problems in a patient who is already hyperkalemic.

150. a. A patient with reactive airway disease would be a candidate for having an increased expiratory phase set on the ventilator. A normal I:E is 1.2, but a reactive airway disease patient may require a 1:3 to allow for exhalation. Without increasing the E time, the patient may experience breath-stacking and increased intrathoracic pressure.

Scoring

Evaluate how you did on this practice exam by first finding the number of questions you answered correctly. Only the number of correct answers is important—questions you skipped or answered incorrectly do not count against your score. Your goal should be a score greater than 80%. The NREMT exam is now computer adaptive and therefore there is no minimum score, just a measure of competency.

Use your scores in conjunction with the LearningExpress Test Preparation System in Chapter 2 of this book to help devise a study plan. You should plan to spend more time on the topics that correspond to the questions you found hardest, and less time on the topics in which you performed well.

Much more important than your overall score, for now, is how you did on each of the topics tested by the exam. You need to diagnose your strengths and weaknesses so that you can concentrate your efforts as you prepare. The question types are mixed in the practice exam, so in order to tell where your strengths and weaknesses lie, you will need to compare your answer sheet with the following table that shows the topic for each question.

PARAMEDIC PRACTICE EXAM 3 DIAGNOSTIC SCORING CHART	
TOPIC	QUESTION #
Airway, Respiration, and Ventilation	29, 30, 31, 32, 34, 38, 41, 42, 43, 45, 46, 47, 48, 50, 51, 72, 86, 94, 95, 105, 106, 107, 113, 118, 150
Cardiology and Resuscitation	2, 3, 5, 11, 19, 22, 24, 49, 58, 59, 60, 61, 63, 64, 65, 66, 68, 69, 70, 71, 75, 76, 77, 78, 79, 80, 81, 114, 145, 146, 147, 148
Trauma	7, 8, 9, 10, 12, 13, 14, 15, 26, 28, 33, 53, 54, 88, 89, 90, 91, 92, 115, 116, 117, 119, 123, 131, 132, 139, 142, 144
Medical/Obstetrics/Gynecology	6, 17, 18, 20, 21, 23, 25, 27, 35, 36, 37, 39, 40, 44, 52, 55, 56, 57, 73, 82, 83, 84, 85, 87, 93, 97, 98, 99, 100, 101, 102, 103, 104, 108, 120, 121, 122, 124, 125, 126, 127, 128, 129, 130
EMS Operations	1, 4, 16, 62, 67, 74, 96, 109, 110, 111, 112, 133, 134, 135, 136, 137, 138, 140, 141, 143, 149

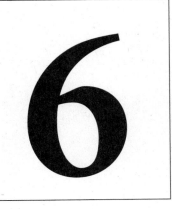

PARAMEDIC PRACTICE EXAM 4

CHAPTER SUMMARY

This is the fourth of five practice exams in this book based on the NREMT EMT-Paramedic/Paramedic written exam. Using all of your experience and strategies that you gained from the other three practice exams, take this exam to see how far you have come since your first one.

Although this is the fourth practice exam in this book, it is not designed to be any harder than the other three. It is simply another representation of what you might find on the real test. There should not be anything here to surprise you. Because you have worked hard taking practice tests, you will be prepared and you will not be surprised.

1.	ⓐ	ⓑ	ⓒ	ⓓ
2.	ⓐ	ⓑ	ⓒ	ⓓ
3.	ⓐ	ⓑ	ⓒ	ⓓ
4.	ⓐ	ⓑ	ⓒ	ⓓ
5.	ⓐ	ⓑ	ⓒ	ⓓ
6.	ⓐ	ⓑ	ⓒ	ⓓ
7.	ⓐ	ⓑ	ⓒ	ⓓ
8.	ⓐ	ⓑ	ⓒ	ⓓ
9.	ⓐ	ⓑ	ⓒ	ⓓ
10.	ⓐ	ⓑ	ⓒ	ⓓ
11.	ⓐ	ⓑ	ⓒ	ⓓ
12.	ⓐ	ⓑ	ⓒ	ⓓ
13.	ⓐ	ⓑ	ⓒ	ⓓ
14.	ⓐ	ⓑ	ⓒ	ⓓ
15.	ⓐ	ⓑ	ⓒ	ⓓ
16.	ⓐ	ⓑ	ⓒ	ⓓ
17.	ⓐ	ⓑ	ⓒ	ⓓ
18.	ⓐ	ⓑ	ⓒ	ⓓ
19.	ⓐ	ⓑ	ⓒ	ⓓ
20.	ⓐ	ⓑ	ⓒ	ⓓ
21.	ⓐ	ⓑ	ⓒ	ⓓ
22.	ⓐ	ⓑ	ⓒ	ⓓ
23.	ⓐ	ⓑ	ⓒ	ⓓ
24.	ⓐ	ⓑ	ⓒ	ⓓ
25.	ⓐ	ⓑ	ⓒ	ⓓ
26.	ⓐ	ⓑ	ⓒ	ⓓ
27.	ⓐ	ⓑ	ⓒ	ⓓ
28.	ⓐ	ⓑ	ⓒ	ⓓ
29.	ⓐ	ⓑ	ⓒ	ⓓ
30.	ⓐ	ⓑ	ⓒ	ⓓ
31.	ⓐ	ⓑ	ⓒ	ⓓ
32.	ⓐ	ⓑ	ⓒ	ⓓ
33.	ⓐ	ⓑ	ⓒ	ⓓ
34.	ⓐ	ⓑ	ⓒ	ⓓ
35.	ⓐ	ⓑ	ⓒ	ⓓ
36.	ⓐ	ⓑ	ⓒ	ⓓ
37.	ⓐ	ⓑ	ⓒ	ⓓ
38.	ⓐ	ⓑ	ⓒ	ⓓ
39.	ⓐ	ⓑ	ⓒ	ⓓ
40.	ⓐ	ⓑ	ⓒ	ⓓ
41.	ⓐ	ⓑ	ⓒ	ⓓ
42.	ⓐ	ⓑ	ⓒ	ⓓ
43.	ⓐ	ⓑ	ⓒ	ⓓ
44.	ⓐ	ⓑ	ⓒ	ⓓ
45.	ⓐ	ⓑ	ⓒ	ⓓ
46.	ⓐ	ⓑ	ⓒ	ⓓ
47.	ⓐ	ⓑ	ⓒ	ⓓ
48.	ⓐ	ⓑ	ⓒ	ⓓ
49.	ⓐ	ⓑ	ⓒ	ⓓ
50.	ⓐ	ⓑ	ⓒ	ⓓ

51.	ⓐ	ⓑ	ⓒ	ⓓ
52.	ⓐ	ⓑ	ⓒ	ⓓ
53.	ⓐ	ⓑ	ⓒ	ⓓ
54.	ⓐ	ⓑ	ⓒ	ⓓ
55.	ⓐ	ⓑ	ⓒ	ⓓ
56.	ⓐ	ⓑ	ⓒ	ⓓ
57.	ⓐ	ⓑ	ⓒ	ⓓ
58.	ⓐ	ⓑ	ⓒ	ⓓ
59.	ⓐ	ⓑ	ⓒ	ⓓ
60.	ⓐ	ⓑ	ⓒ	ⓓ
61.	ⓐ	ⓑ	ⓒ	ⓓ
62.	ⓐ	ⓑ	ⓒ	ⓓ
63.	ⓐ	ⓑ	ⓒ	ⓓ
64.	ⓐ	ⓑ	ⓒ	ⓓ
65.	ⓐ	ⓑ	ⓒ	ⓓ
66.	ⓐ	ⓑ	ⓒ	ⓓ
67.	ⓐ	ⓑ	ⓒ	ⓓ
68.	ⓐ	ⓑ	ⓒ	ⓓ
69.	ⓐ	ⓑ	ⓒ	ⓓ
70.	ⓐ	ⓑ	ⓒ	ⓓ
71.	ⓐ	ⓑ	ⓒ	ⓓ
72.	ⓐ	ⓑ	ⓒ	ⓓ
73.	ⓐ	ⓑ	ⓒ	ⓓ
74.	ⓐ	ⓑ	ⓒ	ⓓ
75.	ⓐ	ⓑ	ⓒ	ⓓ
76.	ⓐ	ⓑ	ⓒ	ⓓ
77.	ⓐ	ⓑ	ⓒ	ⓓ
78.	ⓐ	ⓑ	ⓒ	ⓓ
79.	ⓐ	ⓑ	ⓒ	ⓓ
80.	ⓐ	ⓑ	ⓒ	ⓓ
81.	ⓐ	ⓑ	ⓒ	ⓓ
82.	ⓐ	ⓑ	ⓒ	ⓓ
83.	ⓐ	ⓑ	ⓒ	ⓓ
84.	ⓐ	ⓑ	ⓒ	ⓓ
85.	ⓐ	ⓑ	ⓒ	ⓓ
86.	ⓐ	ⓑ	ⓒ	ⓓ
87.	ⓐ	ⓑ	ⓒ	ⓓ
88.	ⓐ	ⓑ	ⓒ	ⓓ
89.	ⓐ	ⓑ	ⓒ	ⓓ
90.	ⓐ	ⓑ	ⓒ	ⓓ
91.	ⓐ	ⓑ	ⓒ	ⓓ
92.	ⓐ	ⓑ	ⓒ	ⓓ
93.	ⓐ	ⓑ	ⓒ	ⓓ
94.	ⓐ	ⓑ	ⓒ	ⓓ
95.	ⓐ	ⓑ	ⓒ	ⓓ
96.	ⓐ	ⓑ	ⓒ	ⓓ
97.	ⓐ	ⓑ	ⓒ	ⓓ
98.	ⓐ	ⓑ	ⓒ	ⓓ
99.	ⓐ	ⓑ	ⓒ	ⓓ
100.	ⓐ	ⓑ	ⓒ	ⓓ

101.	ⓐ	ⓑ	ⓒ	ⓓ
102.	ⓐ	ⓑ	ⓒ	ⓓ
103.	ⓐ	ⓑ	ⓒ	ⓓ
104.	ⓐ	ⓑ	ⓒ	ⓓ
105.	ⓐ	ⓑ	ⓒ	ⓓ
106.	ⓐ	ⓑ	ⓒ	ⓓ
107.	ⓐ	ⓑ	ⓒ	ⓓ
108.	ⓐ	ⓑ	ⓒ	ⓓ
109.	ⓐ	ⓑ	ⓒ	ⓓ
110.	ⓐ	ⓑ	ⓒ	ⓓ
111.	ⓐ	ⓑ	ⓒ	ⓓ
112.	ⓐ	ⓑ	ⓒ	ⓓ
113.	ⓐ	ⓑ	ⓒ	ⓓ
114.	ⓐ	ⓑ	ⓒ	ⓓ
115.	ⓐ	ⓑ	ⓒ	ⓓ
116.	ⓐ	ⓑ	ⓒ	ⓓ
117.	ⓐ	ⓑ	ⓒ	ⓓ
118.	ⓐ	ⓑ	ⓒ	ⓓ
119.	ⓐ	ⓑ	ⓒ	ⓓ
120.	ⓐ	ⓑ	ⓒ	ⓓ
121.	ⓐ	ⓑ	ⓒ	ⓓ
122.	ⓐ	ⓑ	ⓒ	ⓓ
123.	ⓐ	ⓑ	ⓒ	ⓓ
124.	ⓐ	ⓑ	ⓒ	ⓓ
125.	ⓐ	ⓑ	ⓒ	ⓓ
126.	ⓐ	ⓑ	ⓒ	ⓓ
127.	ⓐ	ⓑ	ⓒ	ⓓ
128.	ⓐ	ⓑ	ⓒ	ⓓ
129.	ⓐ	ⓑ	ⓒ	ⓓ
130.	ⓐ	ⓑ	ⓒ	ⓓ
131.	ⓐ	ⓑ	ⓒ	ⓓ
132.	ⓐ	ⓑ	ⓒ	ⓓ
133.	ⓐ	ⓑ	ⓒ	ⓓ
134.	ⓐ	ⓑ	ⓒ	ⓓ
135.	ⓐ	ⓑ	ⓒ	ⓓ
136.	ⓐ	ⓑ	ⓒ	ⓓ
137.	ⓐ	ⓑ	ⓒ	ⓓ
138.	ⓐ	ⓑ	ⓒ	ⓓ
139.	ⓐ	ⓑ	ⓒ	ⓓ
140.	ⓐ	ⓑ	ⓒ	ⓓ
141.	ⓐ	ⓑ	ⓒ	ⓓ
142.	ⓐ	ⓑ	ⓒ	ⓓ
143.	ⓐ	ⓑ	ⓒ	ⓓ
144.	ⓐ	ⓑ	ⓒ	ⓓ
145.	ⓐ	ⓑ	ⓒ	ⓓ
146.	ⓐ	ⓑ	ⓒ	ⓓ
147.	ⓐ	ⓑ	ⓒ	ⓓ
148.	ⓐ	ⓑ	ⓒ	ⓓ
149.	ⓐ	ⓑ	ⓒ	ⓓ
150.	ⓐ	ⓑ	ⓒ	ⓓ

Paramedic Exam 4

Answer questions 1–4 based on the following information.

You respond to a shortness-of-breath call. Upon arrival, you find the first responders placing a 70-year-old male patient on a nonrebreather mask and running the oxygen flowmeter at 15 lpm. Family members state that the patient came back from the store approximately 45 minutes ago complaining of moderate respiratory distress. He has a history of "some sort of lung disease," for which he uses an inhaler. The family does not know what type of medication the patient is taking. There is no history of fever or recent illness.

You observe that the patient is cyanotic. The oxygen reservoir on the mask does not appear to collapse, even though the liter flow is set correctly. Although he is sitting on the edge of the bed, his eyes are closed and he does not respond to verbal commands. There is accessory muscle use evident with intercostal muscle retractions.

His breath sounds are diminished in all fields and absent in both bases. Faint expiratory wheezing is auscultated at only the apices. His heart rate is 140 BPM, respiratory rate 42 breaths per minute, and blood pressure 106/72 mmHg. The pulse oximeter registers an SpO_2 of 75%. The rest of his physical exam is unremarkable.

1. Based on the information given, what might be a suspected assessment?
   a. toxic inhalation
   b. emphysema
   c. foreign-body obstruction
   d. pneumonia

2. Of the following options, what would be your initial priority in managing this patient's condition?
   a. Get additional medical history from the family.
   b. Instruct first responders to reduce the liter flow from 15 to 10 lpm to allow the reservoir to collapse.
   c. Instruct first responders to assist the patient's ventilations with a BVM and 100% oxygen.
   d. Begin an IV of normal saline.

3. What equipment might you consider first for ventilating this patient?
   a. bag-valve mask
   b. nasal tracheal intubation
   c. CPAP
   d. oropharyngeal airway

4. Which of the following medications may be used in the management of this patient's condition?
   a. morphine sulfate
   b. albuterol
   c. adenosine
   d. epinephrine

5. When using the OPQRST mnemonic to assess a patient's pain, you would assess the R portion of the mnemonic by asking which of the following questions?
   a. "When did it start hurting you?"
   b. "Does the pain move anywhere?"
   c. "What makes it feel better?"
   d. "Does the pain feel sharp or dull?"

6. Which set of signs and symptoms is characteristic of a patient in compensated shock?

a. lethargy, confusion, normal to slightly elevated pulse and blood pressure, cool skin, and delayed capillary refill

b. coma; very low pulse and blood pressure; and pale, cold, and clammy skin with delayed capillary refill time

c. lapsing into unconsciousness, moderately elevated pulse and blood pressure, mottling of extremities, and cyanosis around lips

d. unconsciousness, bradycardia, dropping blood pressure, cold extremities, delayed capillary refill, and absent radial pulses

7. A driver who follows a down-and-under pathway of injury after a collision is most likely to have which type of injury?

a. fractured ribs

b. ruptured diaphragm

c. fractured femur

d. lacerated liver or spleen

8. The paper bag effect occurs when the occupant of a car takes a deep breath just before a collision, resulting in which of the following injuries?

a. pneumothorax

b. pulmonary embolism

c. shearing of the aorta

d. lung laceration

9. Where is a conscious adult who falls a distance of 20 feet most likely to land?

a. head

b. hands

c. back

d. feet

10. Your patient, a middle-aged female, is a pedestrian struck by a car. She opens her eyes only in response to pain and makes no verbal response; her best motor response is withdrawal in response to pain. What is the Glasgow Coma Scale score for this patient?

a. 3

b. 5

c. 7

d. 9

11. Your patient, the victim of an assault, is experiencing malocclusion and numbness to the chin. There is also a suspected nasal fracture, and significant facial bleeding and bruising. What treatment should you apply for this patient?

a. Secure the airway with a nasopharyngeal airway, control bleeding, and transport with the patient sitting upright.

b. Secure the cervical spine, control the airway (but avoid the use of a nasopharyngeal airway), control bleeding, and transport.

c. Treat for signs and symptoms of shock, control the airway with nasal intubation and suction, and transport.

d. Secure the cervical spine, attach ECG monitor, apply PASG, and control the airway (but avoid the use of a nasopharyngeal airway).

12. The presence of marked purplish-red raccoon eyes on a patient in the prehospital environment should lead you to suspect which of the following?

a. sinus injury

b. recent cervical spine trauma

c. a significant mechanism of injury

d. significant previous head injury

13. Your patient is a middle-aged female who has been in a car accident. Because the initial assessment showed no immediate life threats, you are now treating her most serious injuries, which include a suspected broken femur and kneecap. After stabilizing the injured leg and rechecking the pulse, motor responses, and sensation, you should
   a. repeat the initial assessment.
   b. stabilize the cervical spine.
   c. check the proximal pulse.
   d. apply the PASG and transport.

14. Your patient is a 26-year-old construction worker who has fallen approximately 35 feet and suffered multiple injuries. The Glasgow Coma Scale score is 9, respiratory rate is 32 breaths per minute, respiratory expansion is normal, blood pressure is 100/70 mmHg, and capillary refill is delayed. What score should this patient receive if you are using the Revised Trauma Score?
   a. 15
   b. 13
   c. 10
   d. 9

Answer questions 15–17 based on the following information.

Your unit is dispatched to a single-automobile crash. The patient's car hit a large tree head-on. The patient, a young adult woman, is found conscious and alert but trapped in the car. The air bag deployed, but she denies any head or neck pain. She does complain of hip and left leg pain. After a difficult 20-minute extrication, the patient is finally released from the car. Suddenly your patient's vital signs begin to collapse.

15. This patient is most likely transitioning from which of the following?
   a. decompensated shock to hypovolemic shock
   b. cardiogenic shock to hypovolemic shock
   c. compensated shock to decompensated shock
   d. decompensated shock to compensated shock

16. The patient has a closed fracture of the left ankle and the pelvis is stable. There is no penetrating trauma noted in the chest or abdomen, and the patient denies pregnancy. Which of the following chambers of the PASG should be inflated?
   a. both legs and the abdominal compartment
   b. the right leg and the abdominal compartments
   c. the left leg and the abdominal compartments
   d. None; PASG is not indicated in this patient.

17. You start a large bore IV of normal saline. Which of the following medications should you administer?
   a. lidocaine
   b. morphine
   c. dopamine
   d. None; medication is not indicated.

18. A patient who complains of pain in the left upper abdominal quadrant may be suffering from which of the following?
   a. pancreatitis
   b. appendicitis
   c. hepatitis
   d. diverticulitis

19. The signs of uremia resulting from chronic renal failure include
   a. pale skin, diaphoresis, and edematous extremities.
   b. pasty, yellow skin and wasting of the extremities.
   c. anxiety, delirium, nausea, and hallucinations.
   d. anorexia, watery diarrhea, nausea, and vomiting.

20. Your patient is a 75-year-old man. His wife called EMS because he "has a terrible headache and is very confused." Vital signs are respirations 26 breaths per minute; pulse 78 BPM, and blood pressure 200/120 mmHg. The primary problem you must address is most likely which of the following?
   a. hypertensive emergency
   b. senile dementia
   c. cardiac tamponade
   d. stroke

21. Which assessment findings are consistent with cardiogenic shock in a patient who is suffering a presumed AMI?
   a. RR 26 breaths per minute, BP 100/70 mmHg, and cyanosis
   b. RR 10 breaths per minute, BP 160/100 mmHg, and diaphoresis
   c. RR 36 breaths per minute, BP 90/60 mmHg, and cyanosis
   d. RR 18 breaths per minute, BP 140/90 mmHg, and cool, dry skin

Answer questions 22–25 based on the following information.

You respond to a 41-year-old male who has been injured in an explosion at an illegal chemistry (drug) laboratory. During your assessment, you notice a spinal deformity and a possible closed head injury. Your patient also has ruptured tympanic membranes and sinus injuries.

22. Which of the following is NOT a phase of blast injury?
   a. alpha
   b. primary
   c. secondary
   d. tertiary

23. This patient's sinus injuries most likely occurred during which blast phase?
   a. alpha
   b. primary
   c. secondary
   d. tertiary

24. Your victim has first- and second-degree burns to his face. These are flash burns from the explosion. Witnesses deny that the patient's clothes were on fire. What injury should you suspect?
   a. extensive lung tissue burns
   b. extensive airway burns
   c. aspiration pneumonia
   d. limited airway burns

25. During your assessment, you notice a rigid, very tender abdomen. If this injury occurred in the secondary blast phase, it would be due to which of the following?
   a. thermal burns to the stomach
   b. flying debris and propelled objects
   c. deceleration impact with a hard surface
   d. compression of air-containing organs

26. Your patient is a 27-year-old male who is found unconscious on a bathroom floor. He is not breathing, has pinpoint pupils, and has a fresh puncture wound to his right forearm. He has multiple scars that form a bluish streak over the veins on the back of both hands. This patient is most likely suffering from which of the following?
a. seizure disorder
b. multiple spider bites
c. narcotic overdose
d. anaphylactic shock

27. Your patient is an 84-year-old man with extreme difficulty breathing, apprehension, cyanosis, and diaphoresis. Assessment findings include elevated pulse and blood pressure. Crackles and rhonchi are heard on auscultation. There is no chest pain. For what condition should you treat this patient?
a. right-sided heart failure
b. cardiogenic shock secondary to MI
c. dissecting aortic aneurysm
d. left-sided failure secondary to MI

28. Your female patient has a partial airway obstruction, but has adequate air exchange. You should perform which of the following?
a. Perform the Heimlich maneuver as though a complete airway obstruction exists.
b. Intubate the patient nasally in an attempt to bypass the area of obstruction in the lungs.
c. Monitor the patient closely while she continues trying to clear the airway herself.
d. Intubate the patient orally, administer high flow oxygen, and transport immediately.

29. You are caring for a 77-year-old female who is in moderate respiratory distress. She is sitting in a tripod position with two-word dyspnea. She has a recent cold with increasing dyspnea and a productive cough with yellow sputum. She denies chest pain. She has been smoking cigarettes for the past 40 years. Vital signs are BP 150/80 mmHg, P 100 BPM, and RR 36 breaths per minute and labored. Her skin is cyanotic and she has pitting edema in the legs. You hear expiratory wheezing upon auscultation of the lungs. Her pedal edema is most likely caused by which of the following?
a. left-sided heart failure
b. acute pulmonary edema
c. peripheral vasoconstriction
d. cor pulmonale

30. What is an important disadvantage in using both nasal and oropharyngeal airway adjuncts?
a. They are unable to protect the lower airway from aspiration.
b. They may become obstructed by aspirated material.
c. They can be used only in patients whose gag reflex is intact.
d. They are not made in a wide enough range of sizes to fit all patients.

31. After inserting a blind insertion airway device, what step should you take before inflating the balloon to ensure that the tube is properly positioned?
a. Measure the amount of the device outside the mouth.
b. Hyperventilate the patient with 100% oxygen.
c. Look for chest rise and auscultate the lungs and abdomen.
d. Auscultate in the midaxillary line for only bilateral breath sounds.

32. An endotracheal tube that has been advanced too far is prone to enter which of the following structures?
 a. esophagus
 b. trachea
 c. left main bronchus
 d. right main bronchus

Answer questions 33–38 based on the following information.

You are called to a nursing home and find a bedridden 78-year-old male with insulin-dependent diabetes who is in acute respiratory distress. The staff reports that the patient has been ill for the past few days and has had a persistent productive cough with thick yellow sputum. His blood pressure is 168/72. His respiratory rate is 40 and labored with coarse rhonchi upon auscultation of lung sounds. Lung sounds are absent in the lower third of his lung fields. The patient is also febrile with hot, dry, flushed skin.

33. This patient is most likely suffering from which condition?
 a. chronic bronchitis
 b. right-sided heart failure
 c. emphysema
 d. pneumonia

34. Treatment of this patient should include which of the following medications?
 a. albuterol
 b. methylprednisolone
 c. oxygen
 d. bronchodilators

35. What common infectious disease does this patient's clinical presentation mimic?
 a. meningitis
 b. HIV/AIDS
 c. tuberculosis
 d. hepatitis B

36. What is most likely the cause of his decreased lung sounds?
 a. complications from diabetes mellitus
 b. atelectasis from inactivity
 c. congestive heart failure
 d. pulmonary hypertension

37. If this patient required tracheal suctioning, which of the following steps should be followed?
 a. Suction upon insertion of the suction catheter.
 b. Sterile technique is required for suctioning this patient.
 c. Wearing gloves is the only BSI required.
 d. Hyperventilate the patient only after suctioning.

38. How should this patient be positioned for transport?
 a. high Fowler's position
 b. supine
 c. left-lateral recumbent
 d. prone

39. Prehospital care of an open pneumothorax includes which of the following?
 a. high-flow oxygen, monitoring for signs of tension pneumothorax, and intubation
 b. needle decompression, ventilatory support, and rapid transport
 c. occlusive dressing, high-flow oxygen, and rapid transport
 d. airway maintenance, creation of a one-way valve, and fluid boluses

40. Your patient is an adult female whom you suspect is unconscious as a result of an upper-airway obstruction. You use the head-tilt/chin-lift method to open her airway and then attempt a ventilation, which is unsuccessful. What is the next thing you should do?
   a. Give five thrusts on her abdomen.
   b. Give five chest thrusts on her sternum.
   c. Finger-sweep from cheek to cheek.
   d. Reposition and attempt to ventilate again.

41. Your patient is a 67-year-old male who reports a smoking history of 45 packs per year, frequent respiratory infections, and a chronic cough. He is overweight and has peripheral cyanosis. Auscultation of the chest reveals rhonchi. There is also noticeable jugular vein distention. What disease process should you suspect?
   a. emphysema
   b. status asthmaticus
   c. chronic bronchitis
   d. lung cancer

42. When using a peak flow meter to measure peak expiratory flow, the correct procedure is to perform which of the following?
   a. Ask the patient to inhale deeply, then exhale once as quickly as possible, taking one reading.
   b. Ask the patient to inhale normally and exhale twice, recording the lowest reading.
   c. Ask the patient to inhale and exhale as hard and fast as possible, taking only one reading.
   d. Ask the patient to inhale and exhale twice, as hard as possible, recording the highest reading.

43. What is the correct dosage of methylprednisolone for a patient who is experiencing a severe asthma attack?
   a. 300–500 mg given subcutaneously or intramuscularly
   b. 125–250 mg given via IV or intramuscularly
   c. 275 mg given intramuscularly, followed by 1 gram IM 2 hours later
   d. 200–300 mg, diluted in 2–3 mL normal saline, via nebulizer

44. How should you maintain respiratory isolation when transporting a patient suspected of having tuberculosis?
   a. Have the patient ride alone in the back of the ambulance.
   b. Have the patient wear an oxygen mask while in the unit.
   c. Have EMS personnel wear HEPA- or OSHA-approved particle masks.
   d. Have both patient and personnel wear the appropriate masks.

Answer questions 45–50 based on the following information.

You are called to the home of a 26-year-old male who is having difficulty breathing. Your assessment reveals a pulse rate of 100 BPM with a strong and regular radial pulse, a blood pressure of 132/78 mmHg, and a respiratory rate of 36 breaths per minute with labored respirations and audible wheezes. The patient's skin is pale, moist, and at a normal temperature. He is having difficulty exhaling and says that he has experienced this before. He rates this event as a 9 on a 1–10 severity scale. He states that this event was unprovoked and that he has been having dyspnea for 20–30 minutes.

45. This patient is most likely suffering from which of the following conditions?
   a. pulmonary edema
   b. upper-airway obstruction
   c. asthma
   d. simple pneumothorax

46. Which of the following statements is true regarding this patient's treatment with nebulized steroids?
   a. The treatment provides no immediate relief of the bronchospasm.
   b. The treatment reverses the effects of the bronchospasm in the lungs.
   c. The treatment increases the severity of the bronchospasm.
   d. The treatment may be potentially dangerous due to increased blood pressure.

47. Which of the following medications should be used for the treatment of this patient?
   a. terbutaline sulfate
   b. epinephrine 1:1,000 IM
   c. albuterol via nebulizer
   d. all of the above

48. This patient's respiratory distress is due to which of the following?
   a. increased cardiac preload and afterload
   b. decreased left ventricle stroke volume
   c. constriction of the trachea and bronchi
   d. constriction of the smaller airways

49. This patient's disease is regarded as which of the following?
   a. chronic obstructive pulmonary disease
   b. acute obstructive pulmonary disease
   c. chronic inflammatory disease
   d. acute inflammatory disease

50. This patient's respiratory distress may have been caused by one of several triggers. These triggers include allergens, irritants, and which of the following?
   a. viral infections
   b. hot weather
   c. exercise
   d. bee stings

51. Blood enters the right atrium of the heart through which of the following structures?
   a. tricuspid valve
   b. right ventricle
   c. left pulmonary arteries
   d. superior and inferior vena cava

52. What is the estimated systolic blood pressure of a patient whose carotid pulse is palpable, but the radial and femoral pulses are not?
   a. 45 mmHg
   b. 60 mmHg
   c. 85 mmHg
   d. 100 mmHg

53. Simultaneous palpation of the apical impulse and the carotid pulse allows you to assess the relationship between which of the following?
   a. heart and lungs
   b. central and peripheral circulation
   c. pulse and blood pressure
   d. ventricular contractions and pulse

54. You are starting an IV and your first cannulation attempt is unsuccessful. Where should the second attempt be made?
   a. inferior to the first
   b. superior to the first
   c. on a different limb
   d. in a central vein

55. A two-year-old female presents with lethargy and poor feeding. The parent states that the patient has had a moderate fever for the past seven days, with diarrhea, nausea, and vomiting for the past four days. She presents with pale, cool skin, a pulse rate of 180 BPM, and a respiratory rate of 40 breaths per minute. She cries weakly when a painful stimulus is applied. The ECG shows a rapid narrow complex dysrhythmia. Based upon this information, what is the patient's suspected primary problem?
   a. respiratory distress
   b. respiratory failure
   c. hypoperfusion
   d. dysrhythmia

56. What vasopressor drug is most commonly used to treat cardiogenic shock in the prehospital environment?
   a. norepinephrine
   b. epinephrine
   c. dopamine
   d. dobutamine

57. Your patient has suffered penetrating trauma to the neck and is bleeding profusely from several large vessels. You should perform which of the following?
   a. Apply constant direct pressure over the clavicle.
   b. Apply an occlusive dressing, then apply pressure.
   c. Clamp the injured vessels and apply sterile plastic.
   d. Tamponade the vessels with gauze and 4×4s.

58. The signs and symptoms of cerebral hemorrhage include
   a. disorientation and confusion, decreased pulse and blood pressure, and cyanosis.
   b. transient loss of consciousness, headache, drowsiness, nausea, and vomiting.
   c. leakage of cerebrospinal fluid, headache, and bleeding from the nose or ears.
   d. headache, Battle's sign, confusion, lethargy, and rapid loss of consciousness.

59. Which statement about hypoglycemia is correct?
   a. Hypoglycemia may occur in nondiabetic patients, especially in chronic alcoholics.
   b. In nondiabetics, hypoglycemia usually results from overeating and too much exercise.
   c. Signs and symptoms of hypoglycemia are slow in onset and develop over several hours.
   d. In late stages of hypoglycemia, the patient may complain of extreme hunger and thirst.

60. Myocardial infarction may go unrecognized in elderly patients. Why is this true?
   a. They tend to have abnormal ECGs even in the presence of an AMI.
   b. They take prescription nitroglycerin to relieve their symptoms.
   c. They are not able to describe their symptoms clearly to the doctor.
   d. They lack typical symptoms such as frequent chest pain or discomfort.

61. Blood flows from the pulmonary veins into which structure?
   a. left atrium of the heart
   b. right atrium of the heart
   c. capillaries of the lungs
   d. right ventricle of the heart

62. A 12-year-old unconscious male is being brought to the edge of the pool by two life-guards. He is apneic. How would you establish his airway?
a. manual cervical spine precautions, head-tilt/chin-lift
b. manual cervical spine precautions, modified jaw thrust
c. Either is appropriate.
d. Neither is appropriate.

63. What is the effect of parasympathetic stimulation on the heart?
a. an increased heart rate and increased stroke volume
b. a decreased heart rate and increased stroke volume
c. an increased heart rate and decreased stroke volume
d. a decreased heart rate and decreased stroke volume

64. Unilateral wheezing in a 14-month-old child is suggestive of which of the following?
a. asthma
b. aspiration of a foreign body
c. heart failure
d. croup

65. What does a normal P-R interval on an ECG recording indicate?
a. The interventricular septum has been depolarized, and the impulse is now in the AV node.
b. The right and left ventricles have depolarized, sending the impulse to the Purkinje fibers.
c. The ventricular myocardial cells have repolarized during the last part of ventricular systole.
d. The electrical impulse has been successfully conducted through the atria and the AV node.

66. What does a QRS complex that is longer than 0.12 seconds or bizarre in shape indicate?
a. an artifact present on the ECG tracing
b. a conduction abnormality in the ventricles
c. a pacemaker abnormality in the AV node
d. a conduction abnormality in the atria

67. Figure 6.1 indicates which of the following rhythms?
a. junctional escape
b. second-degree heart block, Mobitz type I
c. 60 cycle
d. idioventricular

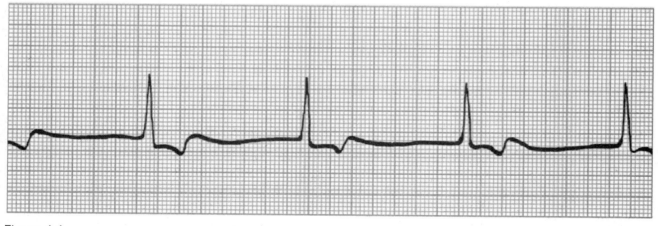

Figure 6.1

68. What is the first treatment for a symptomatic patient with atrial fibrillation with a sustained ventricular rate greater than 150 beats per minute?
   a. vagal or valsalva maneuvers
   b. immediate cardioversion
   c. administration of adenosine
   d. administration of lidocaine

69. Which of the following locations is the most common area of cardiac infarct?
   a. anterior wall
   b. inferior wall
   c. apical wall
   d. medial wall

70. A 50 kg child is apneic and pulseless. The monitor reveals ventricular fibrillation. CPR is in progress. Management of the child will include an initial defibrillation of which of the following?
   a. 25 joules
   b. 50 joules
   c. 100 joules
   d. 200 joules

71. A five-year-old patient weighing 18.2 kg was struck by a car. He is hypotensive and tachycardic. You successfully start an IV in the patient's left antecubital vein. You should infuse which of the following?
   a. 260 mL of NS as a bolus
   b. 360 mL of D_5W as a drip
   c. 800 mL of NS as a bolus
   d. 360 mL of NS as a bolus

72. A patient with a suspected MI but without respiratory compromise should receive oxygen by what rate and delivery device?
   a. 3–4 L/min. by nasal cannula
   b. 5–10 L/min. by simple face mask
   c. 10–15 L/min. by nonrebreather mask
   d. 15–20 L/min. by bag-valve mask

73. Which of the following factors would exclude a patient from receiving thrombolytic therapy after an AMI?
   a. The patient is less than 75 years old.
   b. The chest pain persists after nitroglycerin.
   c. The chest pain lasts longer than 30 minutes.
   d. He or she has had recent ulcer or gastrointestinal bleeding.

74. Which of the following features distinguishes dissecting aortic aneurysm from acute myocardial infarction?
   a. The pain of dissecting aortic aneurysm is severe from the outset.
   b. The pain of dissecting aortic aneurysm usually migrates to the right arm.
   c. Patients with dissecting aortic aneurysm have equal peripheral pulses.
   d. Patients with dissecting aortic aneurysm show signs of pericardial tamponade.

75. What is the prehospital treatment for patients with suspected deep venous thrombosis?
   a. treatment for shock, including oxygen and PASG
   b. administration of nitroglycerin and heparin
   c. initiation of thrombolytic therapy to control the clot
   d. immobilization and elevation of the extremity

76. The presence of delta waves on an ECG is indicative of which of the following?
    a. acute myocardial infarction
    b. new bundle branch block
    c. Wolff-Parkinson-White syndrome
    d. paroxysmal junctional tachycardia

77. Your patient is a 47-year-old male who is experiencing paroxysmal junctional tachycardia. He called EMS because of a sensation of palpitations and lightheadedness. There is no previous history of heart disease. The ventricular rate is approximately 130 beats per minute, BP is 110/70 mmHg, and RR 32 breaths per minute and shallow. What should you do?
    a. Do nothing, as this dysrhythmia is usually well tolerated.
    b. Attempt vagal maneuvers to slow the heart rate down.
    c. Administer 6 mg adenosine by rapid IV bolus.
    d. Attempt synchronized cardioversion with 50 joules.

78. Which of the following features is common to all dysrhythmias that originate in the AV junction?
    a. inverted P waves, shortened P-R interval, normal duration of QRS complex
    b. absent P waves with no P-R interval and prolonged QRS complex
    c. upright P waves, normal P-R interval, normal duration of QRS complex
    d. P waves change from beat to beat or disappear entirely, normal QRS complex

79. A three-year-old male presents with a rapid narrow complex tachycardia with a rate of 260 BPM. He is alert, clings to his parent, and has a strong pulse. How should this patient be treated?
    a. Do nothing, since tachycardia in children is usually well tolerated.
    b. Administer a 20 mL/kg fluid challenge, since this is a shock condition.
    c. Administer adenosine, since this is a stable SVT.
    d. Cardiovert the patient, since this is an unstable SVT.

80. Which of the following statements regarding airway management in the pediatric patient is correct?
    a. The curved blade is preferred in infants and children.
    b. The narrowest diameter of the airway in infants and children is just below the glottic opening.
    c. Cuffed endotracheal tubes should be used in children under the age of eight years.
    d. A 4.0 mm endotracheal tube is recommended for an 18-month-old child.

81. Anxiety may be best defined as which of the following?
    a. a general feeling of uneasiness
    b. an unconscious reaction to a stressor
    c. a factor or event that causes stress
    d. regulation of involuntary movement

Answer questions 82–84 based on the following information.

You respond to a 17-year-old female found unconscious in her backyard by her parents. She has a newly developing skin rash on her right arm and is having difficulty breathing. You note that she is wheezing. Her parents state that she has no history of respiratory problems or other medical disorders.

82. Which of the following is a possible cause of her condition?
   a. anaphylaxis
   b. febrile seizures
   c. status asthmaticus
   d. epiglottitis

83. What is the first step in managing this patient?
   a. Administer IM diphenhydramine.
   b. Give 2 liters of oxygen via NC.
   c. Aggressively manage the airway.
   d. Administer morphine sulfate.

84. The next step in treating this patient is to start a normal saline or lactated Ringer's IV solution and to give which of the following medications?
   a. epinephrine
   b. diphenhydramine
   c. albuterol
   d. morphine sulfate

85. You respond to a scene where a 50 kg child has lost consciousness. The cardiac monitor displays a narrow QRS tachycardia at a rate of 200 beats/minute. A weak pulse is present and the blood pressure is 80/60. Capillary refill is delayed. Oxygen is being administered and an IV has been established. Initial management of this patient will include which of the following?
   a. synchronized countershock with 25 joules
   b. synchronized countershock with 50 joules
   c. unsynchronized countershock with 100 joules
   d. unsynchronized countershock with 200 joules

86. A 72-year-old male is found unconscious in his front yard after working in the yard for five hours without a break. He is tachycardic with hot, dry skin and shallow respirations. Management should include which of the following procedures?
   a. administering furosemide to increase the functioning of the kidneys
   b. administering high-flow oxygen
   c. establishing an IV at TKO rate
   d. preserving body heat to reduce chances of a seizure

87. Before using nitrous oxide for a chest-injury patient, you should exclude the possibility that the patient has which of the following injuries?
   a. cervical spine injury
   b. flail chest
   c. pericardial tamponade
   d. pneumothorax

88. Your patient is a 26-year-old male with a mid-shaft femur fracture and no other apparent injuries. The patient is alert and oriented, and all vital signs are normal. The best way to immobilize this fracture is to use which of the following devices?
   a. PASG/MAST
   b. long spine board
   c. traction splint
   d. softly padded board

89. An adult with burns over the front of both arms and the chest is burned over what percentage of her body surface area (BSA)?
   a. 9%
   b. 13%
   c. 18%
   d. 27%

90. How will the skin over a second-degree burn appear?
   a. bright red
   b. mottled red
   c. pearly white
   d. charred black

91. Which patient is most likely to need burn center care versus trauma center care?
   a. female, age 34, second-degree burn over 10% of BSA
   b. male, age 46, third-degree burn over a small area of the back
   c. female, age 52, second-degree burns to face and right hand
   d. male, age 27, second-degree burn over entire left arm excluding hand

92. Prehospital care for a patient who has moderate to severe burns includes which of the following?
   a. wet dressings, one IV line held at a TKO rate, IV antibiotics
   b. wet dressings, two IV lines with large-bore catheters
   c. dry sterile dressings, one IV line held at a TKO rate, epinephrine 1:1,000
   d. dry sterile dressings, two IV lines with large-bore catheters with appropriate fluid bolus

93. How does a patient who experienced a seizure, rather than a period of syncope, usually report the episode?
   a. It started when she was standing up.
   b. It happened without any warning.
   c. It was associated with bradycardia.
   d. It lasted only two to three minutes.

94. What is included in the management of a patient in a postictal state?
   a. having the patient sit up, administering high-flow oxygen, and transporting immediately
   b. placing the patient in shock position and treating for signs and symptoms of shock
   c. moving obstacles away from the patient, or moving him or her to a safe location
   d. placing the patient in a recumbent position and administering supplemental oxygen

95. General management for a patient with altered mental status should include which of the following procedures?
a. providing low-flow oxygen
b. applying a 12-lead ECG
c. determining blood glucose levels
d. administering dextrose routinely

96. What are the two most common causes of severe anaphylaxis?
a. shellfish and roasted peanuts
b. aspirin and synthetic opiates
c. egg whites and sesame seeds
d. penicillin and insect bites/stings

97. A 72-year-old male is complaining of difficulty breathing. His ECG shows a rate of 44 with corresponding pulses, a P-R interval of 0.18, and normal RR intervals. Vitals are blood pressure 92/56 and respirations 32. The patient also states that he feels very nauseated and dizzy. Treatment for this patient should include which of the following?
a. atropine 0.5 mg
b. epinephrine 1:1,000 0.3 mg
c. epinephrine 1:10,000 1 mg
d. isuprel 2–10 mcg/min.

98. A 52-year-old male patient is experiencing chest palpitations and shortness of breath. Vitals are blood pressure 116/64, pulse 180 bpm and regular, and respirations 36. ECG shows a narrow complex rhythm at a rate of 200 and no discernible P waves. Which of the following regimens is indicated for this patient?
a. IV, O_2, adenosine 6 mg
b. IV, O_2, atropine 0.5 mg
c. IV, O_2, lidocaine 1.5 mg/kg
d. IV, O_2, verapamil 2.5 mg

99. A 58-year-old patient is experiencing shortness of breath. ECG shows a sinus tachycardia at 126. Pulse is weak and blood pressure is 82/52. Which medication and dose would be most appropriate for this patient?
a. dopamine 5–10 mcg/kg/min.
b. furosemide 40 mg
c. morphine sulfate 5 mg
d. nitroglycerin 0.4 mg SL

100. Which finding is helpful in distinguishing poisoning by spider venom from an acute abdominal condition?
a. abdominal rigidity with no palpable tenderness
b. right-lower-quadrant pain in the absence of fever
c. diaphoresis accompanied by chills and fever
d. the presence of multiple bite marks on the stomach

101. Early symptoms of overdose of tricyclic antidepressants include
a. tachycardia and a wide QRS complex.
b. nausea, vomiting, and severe diarrhea.
c. psychosis and bizarre behavioral changes.
d. altered mental status and slurred speech.

102. Which of the following patient scenarios is the typical profile for a victim of classic heat stroke?
a. a healthy young adult who has been exercising in hot, humid weather
b. someone sweating profusely and drinking large amounts of water without salt
c. an elderly person with chronic illness who is confined to a hot room
d. an infant who is exposed to overly high ambient temperatures indoors

103. Which statement about suicide is correct?
   a. People who talk about suicide rarely attempt it by deadly means.
   b. Suicidal patients are mentally ill and require institutionalization.
   c. The suicide rate is lowest during holiday seasons or birthdays.
   d. There is a high correlation between suicide attempts and alcohol consumption.

Answer questions 104–106 based on the following information.

You respond to a four-year-old female who has taken an unknown quantity of children's aspirin. Upon arrival, you find the patient conscious, crying, and lethargic. Her mother states that she found the child playing in the bathroom. A flavored children's aspirin bottle was found nearby with only a few tablets in it.

104. In this situation, what assumption should you make?
   a. The aspirin bottle was full and treat accordingly.
   b. The child couldn't possibly have taken all the aspirin tablets.
   c. There is a reason to suspect child abuse due to neglect.
   d. Because of new packaging laws, the child is not in danger of overdosing.

105. Children's aspirin is in which of the following classes of medications?
   a. tricyclics
   b. acetaminophen
   c. salicylates
   d. benzodiazepines

106. Correct treatment for this patient may include which of the following?
   a. IV, oxygen, naloxone, and NG tube insertion
   b. IV, oxygen, ECG, and activated charcoal
   c. IV, ECG, sodium bicarbonate, and epinephrine
   d. IV, naloxone, and activated charcoal

107. A 52-year-old female is complaining of chest tightness with radiation to the back. Her ECG shows a sinus tachycardia with multifocal premature ventricular contractions occurring 10 times per minute. Her blood pressure is 112/68, and her heart rate is 96 and irregular. Which of the following medications would be indicated for her condition?
   a. lidocaine
   b. adenosine
   c. magnesium sulfate
   d. nitroglycerine

108. What is the usual pediatric dose of naloxone via IV bolus for a child less than five years old?
   a. 0.01 mg/kg
   b. 0.1 mg/kg
   c. 1 mg
   d. 2 mg

109. You are called to the scene of a possible drowning at a local pool. Upon arrival, you discover that lifeguards have removed the patient from the pool and are performing cardiopulmonary resuscitation since the patient is apneic and pulseless. Upon placing the monitor on the patient, you discover a rapid rhythm at 200 beats per minute, no P waves, and a QRS complex of 0.16. Management should consist of which of the following?
   a. amiodarone 150 mg
   b. cardioversion 100 joules
   c. defibrillation 360 joules
   d. lidocaine 1.5 mg/kg

110. Your patient is seven years old and has a suspected broken arm and numerous bruises. The mother states that the child was hurt when he fell off his bike in the morning. What finding would lead you to suspect that the mother's account of the injuries is not true?
- **a.** multiple fresh bruises on the child's arm and leg
- **b.** the child cries from pain when you palpate
- **c.** the child clings to the mother during transport
- **d.** purplish, yellowish, and greenish bruises

Answer questions 111–113 based on the following information.

You respond to a 25-year-old female who is complaining of vaginal bleeding and abdominal pain. The patient states that she is 33 weeks pregnant and that this is her first pregnancy. She says that when the pain started, it felt like "something was tearing." She denies vaginal bleeding during the pregnancy prior to this event. Upon assessment, you notice what appears to be approximately 500 mL of dark, almost black, blood.

111. From which condition is this patient most likely suffering?
- **a.** abruptio placenta
- **b.** placenta previa
- **c.** uterine rupture
- **d.** eclampsia

112. This condition endangers whose life?
- **a.** the mother only
- **b.** the baby only
- **c.** neither patient
- **d.** both patients

113. In addition to high-flow oxygen and continuous monitoring of the mother's vital signs and the baby's fetal heart tones, you should treat this patient with which of the following?
- **a.** one or two large-bore IVs of normal saline or lactated Ringer's solution
- **b.** one minidrip IV of normal saline and pitocin or terbutaline
- **c.** one minidrip IV and PASG with all compartments inflated
- **d.** Basic life support treatments are all that is needed.

114. Patients with pelvic inflammatory disease often complain of which of the following?
- **a.** diffuse lower-abdominal pain
- **b.** severe vaginal bleeding
- **c.** tearing pain in the uterus
- **d.** itching upon urination

115. The two primary goals of prehospital care of a sexual assault victim are to preserve the victim's privacy and dignity and to perform which of the following?
- **a.** Obtain a complete description of the assault.
- **b.** Collect samples of body fluids from the patient.
- **c.** Preserve all physical evidence for the police.
- **d.** Help the victim bathe and change her clothing.

116. A 24-year-old female is complaining of chest pain and difficulty breathing. She has been up for three days studying for finals and has been taking ephedrine supplements to help her stay awake and alert. She also admits to drinking 12 caffeinated soft drinks in the past day. Vitals are BP 80/40 mmHg; P 180 BPM; carotid; and RR 42 breaths per minute. She is very pale and lethargic. The ECG shows a narrow QRS complex with regular RR intervals and no discernible P or T waves at 200 beats per minute. The best treatment for this patient would include which of the following?
   a. adenosine 6 mg rapid IVP
   b. cardioversion at 100 joules
   c. vagal maneuvers
   d. verapamil 2.5 mg slow IVP

117. Your patient is a 32-year-old woman who reports that she is nine weeks pregnant. She is complaining of severe abdominal pain, slight vaginal bleeding, and shoulder pain. Abdominal examination reveals significant tenderness in the lower right quadrant. The patient is somewhat agitated and tachycardic. You should suspect developing shock resulting from which of the following conditions?
   a. ruptured appendix
   b. abruptio placenta
   c. placenta previa
   d. ectopic pregnancy

118. What is the usual clinical presentation of placenta previa?
   a. tearing pain and dark red bleeding
   b. diffuse abdominal pain and slight bleeding
   c. painless bright red bleeding
   d. elevated blood pressure and diffuse pain

119. Which of the following findings or factors would make you opt for immediate transport of a pregnant woman rather than attempt delivery in the field?
   a. the mother's urge to push
   b. the presence of crowning
   c. meconium-stained amniotic fluid
   d. multiparity with explosive births

120. During a normal delivery, you would suction the infant's mouth and nose just after
   a. the head is out of the vagina.
   b. the entire infant is delivered.
   c. the head and chest are delivered.
   d. you clamp the cord.

121. You are managing a patient with symptomatic bradycardia and multifocal PVCs. Suddenly, your patient slumps unconscious and goes into ventricular fibrillation. You confirm that your patient is pulseless. What is your next action?
   a. Administer lidocaine 1.5 mg/kg.
   b. Begin CPR.
   c. Cardiovert at 200 joules.
   d. Defibrillate at 360 joules.

122. What is the correct method to stimulate respirations in a neonate?
   a. Hold it by the feet while you slap the buttocks.
   b. Flick the soles of the feet and rub the back.
   c. Let the cool air cause it to shiver a little.
   d. Rub the head but avoid touching the fontanel.

123. What is the greatest concern when a person experiences blunt force trauma to the head?
a. It can interrupt the integrity of the blood brain barrier.
b. It can cause a significant increase in intracranial pressure.
c. It can cause significant ringing in the ears.
d. It can lacerate the scalp, causing bleeding.

Answer questions 124–127 based on the following information.

You respond to a 19-year-old female who is 25 weeks pregnant and is complaining of a severe headache and blurred vision. Upon initial assessment, you notice that she has substantial edema, especially in her feet and hands. She states that she has not been under the regular care of a physician during this pregnancy.

124. What abnormality would you expect to see in this patient's vital signs?
a. tachycardia
b. tachypnea
c. hypertension
d. hypotension

125. From which condition is this patient is most likely suffering?
a. eclampsia
b. placenta previa
c. preeclampsia
d. supine-hypotensive disorder

126. Treatment for this patient includes rapid transport without lights and sirens, an IV of normal saline or lactated Ringer's solution, and oxygen. It may also call for the administration of which of the following medications?
a. magnesium sulfate
b. pitocin
c. terbutaline sulfate
d. naloxone

127. If left untreated, this patient's condition may worsen and she may begin to experience which of the following?
a. angina pectoris
b. necrosis of tissues
c. grand mal seizures
d. labor pains

128. You are caring for a 69-year-old AMI patient using online medical control. A bystander, who identifies herself as a physician, looks at the ECG, sees you beginning to administer epinephrine, and requests that you substitute atropine. What should you do?
a. Have the online physician consult directly with the on-scene physician.
b. Follow the directions of the on-scene physician who has assumed care.
c. Ignore the on-scene physician and follow the directions of the online physician.
d. Leave the scene and the patient in the care of the on-scene physician.

129. Bradycardia refers to a heart rate that is less than how many beats per minute?
a. 30
b. 40
c. 50
d. 60

130. Which of the following statements regarding falls among the elderly is most accurate?
a. The elderly have the highest incidence of falls.
b. Fall-related injuries represent the leading cause of accidental death among the elderly.
c. Falls account for the highest percentage of emergency department visits among the elderly.
d. A majority of falls are primarily related to infrapatellar bursitis.

131. In which of the following situations is an EMS provider required to make a report to law enforcement?
   a. suspected sexual assault
   b. alcohol-related trauma
   c. MCV with entrapment
   d. illegal drug possession

132. Which patient may be legally placed in protective custody by the police if he or she refuses treatment?
   a. a competent 85-year-old man who has signed a DNR order at the nursing home
   b. a patient who is drunk and disorderly and who refuses treatment for a head wound
   c. an epileptic patient who has just recovered from a seizure but refuses transport
   d. a diabetic who has just recovered from insulin shock and wants to go home

133. You are dispatched to the home of a dying patient who has signed a do-not-resuscitate order. What should you do?
   a. Contact medical control before providing any patient care.
   b. Give only emotional support to the patient and family members.
   c. Carry out all necessary care since such orders apply only to hospitals.
   d. Leave immediately without providing any care for the patient.

134. Pharmacological management of postpartum hemorrhage may include which of the following?
   a. oxytocin
   b. magnesium sulfate
   c. procainamide
   d. amiodarone

135. You are conducting triage using the START system at a major incident. You encounter a patient who is not breathing. After you position the airway, the patient begins to breathe at a rate of six respirations per minute. Into which category would you now triage this patient?
   a. expectant/deceased
   b. immediate
   c. delayed
   d. minor

136. What are the set of duties and skills that a paramedic is permitted to perform during a medical situation?
   a. primary practice
   b. consent to practice
   c. scope of practice
   d. regional practice

137. For which of the following procedures is it necessary to wear gloves, gown, mask, and protective eyewear?
   a. starting an IV in a moving ambulance
   b. bleeding control with minimal bleeding
   c. assisting with an emergency childbirth
   d. administering an intramuscular injection

138. Which form of hepatitis poses the lowest risk to paramedics?
   a. hepatitis A
   b. hepatitis B
   c. hepatitis C
   d. hepatitis D

139. You are interviewing 87-year-old Mrs. Rodriguez, who called EMS but seems to be having difficulty describing her primary problem. Mrs. Rodriguez speaks in English, but is answering your questions slowly and haltingly. Her 20-year-old grandson is also present. What should you do in an attempt to obtain the necessary information?
   a. Direct your questions to the grandson only, since Mrs. Rodriguez is probably senile.
   b. Ask the grandson to translate for Mrs. Rodriguez since she does not understand you.
   c. Ask questions slowly, clearly, and respectfully, giving Mrs. Rodriguez time to respond.
   d. Stop the interview and ask the grandson to leave the room, then resume questioning.

140. Which of the following is NOT typically a characteristic of an abused elderly person?
   a. wealthy but refuses to give financial assistance to relatives
   b. multiple physical and mental impairments, such as dementia
   c. incontinent, mentally handicapped, and over the age of 65
   d. physically handicapped, over the age of 75, and frail

141. Which of the following is an example of acknowledging and labeling the patient's feelings?
   a. "Stop threatening me. I've never hurt you."
   b. "You seem angry. Do you want to tell me about it?"
   c. "I get angry myself sometimes."
   d. "Anger is a hostile emotion. Let's be more positive."

Answer questions 142–145 based on the following information.

Your ambulance is the first on the scene of a suspected radiation emergency. Dispatch has stated that a box containing radioactive material was found unattended and open in a park. No patients have been identified yet, and the police department is sealing off the area.

142. What are the three principles of safety you should keep in mind as you approach the park?
   a. time, distance, and shielding
   b. distance, crowd control, and decontamination
   c. decontamination, clothing, and eye protection
   d. gloves, eye protection, and shielding

143. If you are asked to set up a staging area for additional responding rescue crews, which of the following would be the best location?
   a. upwind, close visual range, in an open area
   b. downwind, close visual range, in an open area
   c. upwind, no visual range, in a building
   d. downwind, no visual range, in a building

144. In this situation, who has the responsibility for decontamination of patients?
   a. first responding ambulance
   b. first responding fire agency
   c. hazardous materials team
   d. triage and treatment officer

145. Which type of radiation is the most serious?
   a. alpha particles
   b. beta particles
   c. gamma rays
   d. delta rays

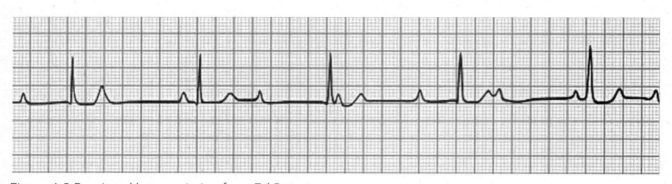

Figure 6.2 Reprinted by permission from Ed Burns.

146. What is the rhythm in Figure 6.2?
   a. sinus bradycardia
   b. junctional escape rhythm
   c. second-degree AV block, Mobitz type II
   d. third-degree AV block

147. Where is the location of the infarct in the 12-lead ECG in Figure 6.3?
   a. septal wall MI
   b. lateral wall MI
   c. inferior-lateral wall MI
   d. anterior wall MI

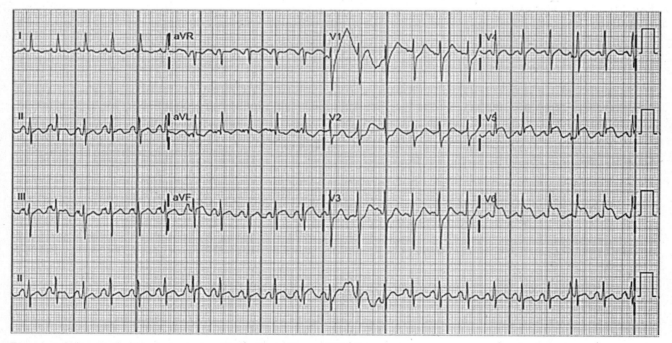

Figure 6.3 Reprinted by permission from Float Nurse (2011).

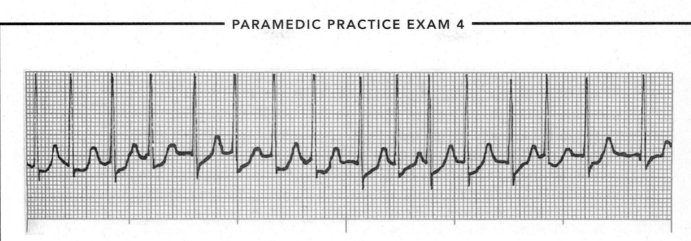

Figure 6.4 Reprinted by permission from Paula Anderson (2004).

148. You respond to a 55-year-old female patient complaining of chest pressure and heart palpitations. The patient's skin is pink, warm, and dry. Her vital signs are a P 160 BPM, BP 104/66 mmHg, RR 24 breaths per minute, blood glucose 92 mg/dl, and oxygen saturation 98%. You have placed the patient on high-flow oxygen and established an IV. Identify the rhythm in Figure 6.4 and the appropriate first-line pharmacological treatment.
  a. ventricular tachycardia treated with 1 mg/kg lidocaine
  b. supraventricular tachycardia with 6 mg adenosine rapid IV push
  c. rapid atrial fibrillation with 0.25 mg/kg of diltiazem slow IV over 2 minutes
  d. sinus tachycardia with no pharmacological intervention required

149. Which of the following is true regarding succinylcholine?
  a. Its effects can be reversed with naloxone.
  b. It causes fasciculations.
  c. It is a nondepolarizing paralytic.
  d. It contains paralytic and sedative properties.

150. Which of the following is true regarding hyperventilation of a patient?
  a. Hyperventilation will increase PCO_2.
  b. Hyperventilation should be used in all patients with increased intracranial pressure.
  c. Hyperventilation will increase intrathoracic pressure, decreasing cardiac preload.
  d. Hyperventilation should be used during cardiac arrest to hyperoxgenate the brain.

Answers

1. b. The timing of the onset, medical history, and physical findings point to emphysema.

2. c. This patient has a decompensated ability to ventilate adequately, as evidenced by the decreased mental status and very poor skin signs. This patient will require aggressive airway management in order to be ventilated.

3. c. The most immediate piece of ventilation equipment to use is CPAP. CPAP eliminates the need for intubation. If CPAP is not available, a bag-valve mask (BVM) would be the next choice. The patient will need preoxygenation before any attempt at intubation. In addition, as implied by the patient's presenting position, he will likely have an intact gag reflex, making insertion of an OPA difficult, if not impossible.

4. b. A beta-agonist like albuterol is indicated in this situation. Morphine sulfate may worsen the patient's condition by potentially depressing respiratory drive. Adenosine is a cardiac medication used to control supraventricular tachycardia. Epinephrine has significant cardiac side effects, especially in older patients.

5. b. In the OPQRST mnemonic, R stands for region and radiation. You should determine if the pain is radiating, referred, or causing any associated problems.

6. a. The signs and symptoms given (lethargy, confusion, normal to slightly elevated pulse and blood pressure, cool skin, and delayed capillary refill) are characteristic of early, or compensated, shock. The single characteristic signaling the change from compensated to uncompensated shock is a drop in blood pressure that remains below normal despite intervention and treatment. You should never wait to see a decrease in BP to decide if shock is present or not, since, early in the shock process, sympathetic stimulation during compensation may result in a slight elevation of the diastolic blood pressure.

7. c. The down-and-under pathway results in injury to the pelvis and legs rather than to the abdominal and thoracic organs. These injuries are caused as the patient's knees strike the lower part of the dashboard; energy forces travel along the femur to the pelvis and maybe even into the lower spine.

8. a. The paper bag effect or paper bag syndrome is thought to be responsible for most pneumothoraces that result from car crashes. During this event, the closed glottis traps pressurized air in the chest. When compression occurs during the crash against the closed glottis, severe damage can occur to the hyperinflated alveoli and bronchioles, resulting in collapse.

9. d. Conscious adults who fall more than three times their height tend to land on their feet; this tends to cause bilateral calcaneus fractures, hip dislocations, and compression fractures of the spinal column.

10. c. Her score is 7: 2 points for pain, 1 point for verbal response, and 4 points for motor response.

11. b. Patients with facial fractures also have suspected spinal trauma and should be immobilized appropriately. Avoid the use of any nasopharyngeal airway manipulations in a patient with facial fractures, as the device could be introduced directly into the brain by perforating through the area of the fracture. Cardiac (ECG) monitoring, pulse oximetry, and other monitoring devices are always appropriate when you have a seriously injured patient. PASG is not indicated in this patient.

12. d. Periorbital ecchymosis, or raccoon eyes, presents as bruises circling around the eyes. It often indicates basal or other skull fracture; however, when seen in the prehospital environment, it suggests significant previous injury because this condition takes time to develop after injury. The earliest finding you would note with a newly developing skull injury is extreme swelling of the soft tissues around each eye that may make it difficult even to open the eyes to check pupils.

13. a. Quickly repeat the initial assessment after every significant intervention. You and your partner have had your attention on her lower extremity for a few minutes, and now you should refocus and repeat an ABC assessment. Cervical immobilization with a collar should be completed prior to treatment of the leg. Proximal pulse check is part of the reassessment survey that occurs immediately after stabilizing and splinting the leg. PASG/MAST is not indicated for this patient.

14. c. The score on the Glasgow Coma Scale translates into 2 points on the Revised Trauma Score; the patient receives 3 points for respiratory rate, 1 point for respiratory expansion, 4 points for blood pressure, and 1 point for delayed capillary refill. The Revised Trauma Score drops the score for respiratory effort and capillary refill. On the Revised Trauma Score, this patient would score 3 points for the GCS, 4 points for their BP, and 3 points for respiratory rate for a total RTS of 10.

15. c. This patient's body is showing signs that it can no longer compensate for the damage done by the traumatic event. In addition, toxic metabolic products may have been trapped in the injured tissues and now are circulating back toward the heart. These toxins may result in cardiac dysrhythmias or cardiac arrest.

16. d. PASG is no longer indicated for routine management of shock patients. If this patient has an unstable pelvis fracture in addition to the presence of shock, PASG could be used as an air splint to assist in stabilizing the fractured pelvis. Because the pelvis is intact, it would be better to rapidly transport her (after full body and cervical spine immobilization) to a well-padded long spine board. Shock can be managed with oxygen, positioning (elevate lower end of long board), rapid transport, and careful fluid administration. You would never inflate only one leg and the abdominal section. Most likely, the garment would not help stabilize the ankle fracture; additional splinting would be required.

17. d. Although your assessment of the pelvis was negative, the mechanism of injury suggests this patient is most likely hemorrhaging internally, resulting in hypovolemic shock. Medications are rarely used in the prehospital management of hypovolemic shock. Your treatment centers around improving oxygenation and prompt transport to the appropriate definitive care facility. Morphine sulfate may help control pain, but its use for this patient is not advisable in the prehospital setting due to the unknown nature of all of her injuries. Dopamine is indicated for cardiogenic shock and is never indicated with uncorrected hypovolemic shock.

18. a. Pain in the left upper quadrant is most often due to pancreatitis, gastritis, or diseases of the left kidney. Appendicitis often results in right-lower-quadrant pain, but the actual location of the area of the appendix that is inflamed may result in left-lower-quadrant or even flank pain. Hepatitis results in dull right-upper-quadrant pain that is independent of the presence of food in the GI tract. Diverticulitis presents much like appendicitis, but it is generally localized to the left lower abdomen.

19. b. Signs of uremia are pasty, yellow skin and thin extremities; urea frost is a late sign. These signs result from jaundice, poor nutrition, and protein loss in the tissues. In extreme cases, the potassium level can be dangerously elevated. Pericardial tamponade, uremic encephalopathy, kidney failure, noncardiac pulmonary edema, severe dyspnea, ascities, neck vein distension, and crackles in the bases may also be seen.

20. a. Although the chief complaint was headache and confusion, it is likely that the primary problem to address is hypertensive crisis. Senile dementia of new onset could have a variety of causes, but in this case, it may be connected to the hypertensive crisis. There is not enough information to determine if elder abuse or cardiac tamponade is present, but it is unlikely in this scenario. Another possibility for this patient is a stroke, but the primary problem to address is prompt management of the hypertensive crisis, which can reduce morbidity.

21. c. In a patient with acute MI, signs of cardiogenic shock result from cardiac insufficiency from decreased coronary artery perfusion due to inadequate pumping of the heart (mainly the left ventricle). The signs and symptoms include low blood pressure; cyanosis or cool, clammy skin; and rapid breathing. Most of these patients have adequate blood volume and vascular system, but have an ineffective pump.

22. a. Blast injury impact is divided into three phases: primary, secondary, and tertiary. The primary phase occurs during the initial air blast and pressure wave. The secondary phase occurs when the patient is hit by debris propelled by the overpressure of the blast wave. The tertiary phase occurs when the victim is thrown away from the blast into the ground or other hard objects.

23. b. During the primary blast, forces from the pressure wave and initial air blast result in compression of air-containing organs such as the sinuses, auditory canals, stomach, lungs, and intestines.

24. d. Often, burns are limited to the oro- and nasopharynx in the upper airway. Worsening stridor or hoarseness indicates that edema is developing, which may lead to airway compromise. Flash burns rarely result in extensive airway or lung tissue burns. Aspiration pneumonia is an infectious process that develops following the introduction of a foreign body into the lungs. Aspiration pneumonia is unlikely in this scenario; if it has occurred, there will be no signs of infection yet.

25. b. Compression of air-containing organs is common in the primary blast phase. Deceleration injuries occur during the tertiary phase and thermal burns can occur during any phase of the blast, depending upon whether the pressure wave is superheated, if flaming objects are striking the patient, or if the patient is thrown into a burning area. A rigid, tender abdomen indicates there are internal injuries under the skin, and not surface injuries to the dermis from burns. This injury was most likely caused by flying debris or propelled objects striking the patient.

26. c. These are the common signs of a narcotic overdose. Pinpoint pupils are characteristic of heroin and narcotic use. A fresh puncture wound over a vein indicates a recent injection site, and bluish scarring over the veins is consistent with the presence of track marks.

27. d. The patient is displaying signs and symptoms of left ventricular failure, which most often occurs secondary to MI. Hypertension and tachycardia is due in part to increased left atrial pressure that is transmitted to the pulmonary vessels. Crackles and rhonchi indicate that pulmonary edema is present. Right-sided failure can lead to left-sided failure, but such a patient generally has dry lungs and dependent edema (usually pedal) as the presenting signs. If the ventricular failure worsens, cardiogenic shock may develop; you will see the systolic pressure drop dramatically (often to less than 80 mmHg) when this occurs. A dissecting aneurysm will present with pain, syncope, stroke, absent or reduced pulses, heart failure, pericardial tamponade, and/or signs of AMI.

28. c. If a patient has a partial airway obstruction but adequate air exchange, allow her to continue her spontaneous efforts to clear the airway (coughing), but monitor her carefully. Your interference may actually worsen the obstruction by making it complete. If air exchange becomes inadequate, treat her as if the obstruction is total by performing the Heimlich, intubation, suction, or other efforts to relieve the obstruction.

29. d. Patients with COPD maintain chronic high levels of CO_2, which may result in pulmonary hypertension and lead to right-sided heart failure, or cor pulmonale.

30. a. Neither the nasopharyngeal nor the oropharyngeal airway is long enough to protect the lower airway from aspirated material. Generally, the presence of vomitus or blood in the airway does not affect their use, since suction is easily performed through and around these devices. Use of the oropharyngeal airway is limited to patients who do not have a gag reflex. The devices come in a wide variety of sizes and styles.

31. c. Regardless of which device you use, confirmation of placement is generally advisable prior to inflation of any balloons on the device by looking for chest rise and fall and listening for breath sounds in the chest and abdomen.

32. d. Because of the anatomical appearance of the distal trachea, it is most common for an ET tube that has been inserted too far to enter the right main bronchus, resulting in atelectasis and insufficiency of the left lung.

33. d. This patient shows signs and symptoms of pneumonia. The fever is the symptom that provides the differential diagnosis between the various choices.

34. c. In addition to oxygen, this patient needs antibiotics.

35. c. Active tuberculosis presents with fever, flu-like symptoms, and productive cough. Meningitis presents with high fever and flulike symptoms, but does not have respiratory involvement. HIV may not have any symptoms, although AIDS can present as a variety of diseases, depending upon which opportunistic disease has caused infection. Hepatitis B will present primarily with GI problems (nausea, vomiting, and pain) and upper-right-quadrant abdominal pain.

36. b. Diabetic patients heal more slowly from pneumonia, but it is not a common disease for them. CHF and pulmonary hypertension would certainly contribute to worsening his signs and symptoms, but the most likely cause of absent or decreased lung sounds in the lower lobes of a sick elderly patient is incomplete expansion and shallow respiration due to inactivity.

37. b. Because tracheal suctioning will be performed on this patient, sterile technique is required. Suction should be performed only upon withdrawal of the catheter. For protection of the rescuer, gloves, eye protection, and face mask should be worn during the procedure. If the patient is being ventilated you should hyperventilate before and after suctioning.

38. a. Position of comfort is always the optimal transport position for nontraumatic patients when the patient is conscious and oriented. To facilitate breathing and maximize efforts, the best position for this patient would be high Fowler's position.

39. c. The steps involved in management of this injury are occlusive dressing, high-flow oxygen, and rapid transport. Intubation is not necessary for each patient. Needle decompression is not necessary unless a tension pneumothorax develops. If dyspnea worsens, open the dressing to relieve some of the pressure that is built up. An IV lifeline should be established but large volume fluid resuscitation should be withheld.

40. d. During the initial resuscitation attempt, the next step after one unsuccessful attempt at ventilation for an unconscious adult patient is to reposition the head and try again. Once you have confirmed obstruction, you do not need to repeat this step again. Blind finger sweeps and abdominal thrusts are no longer recommended. Perform chest compressions at a ratio of 30:2 until the foreign body is removed from the airway.

41. c. The patient's history, signs, and symptoms are consistent with chronic bronchitis. The blue bloater frequently has peripheral edema, cyanosis, and JVD due to right-side heart failure in addition to the respiratory problems. Emphysema patients present with barrel chest and signs of wasting of the extremities.

42. a. The correct procedure is to have the patient inhale deeply and exhale quickly. Some meters ask you to repeat the procedure and average your findings, but you would still have the patient inhale deeply and quickly exhale with each reading.

43. b. The correct dosage and route is 125–250 mg, given via IV or intramuscularly.

44. d. Both the patient and all personnel who come in contact with him or her should wear appropriate masks in order to maintain respiratory isolation. For your own legal protection and for the optimal patient care, you should never transport a patient unattended in your unit.

45. c. This patient shows the clinical symptoms of asthma. Due to the repeat nature of this episode, it is unlikely that this is pulmonary edema, upper-airway obstruction, or simple pneumothorax. If he were suffering from pulmonary edema, you would also expect hemoptysis. A spontaneous (or simple) pneumothorax would also present with a sudden onset, but would most likely not also have wheezing or a history of recurrence.

46. a. Nebulized steroids would provide no immediate relief of this patient's bronchospasm, as they will not prevent or lessen attacks in progress. Steroid therapy is useful as a long-term suppressive treatment.

47. d. Any of these medications can be used to treat this patient.

48. d. Constriction of the smaller airways is causing air to be trapped in the alveoli.

49. c. Asthma is regarded as a chronic inflammatory disease. Chronic obstructive pulmonary diseases commonly include emphysema and chronic bronchitis.

50. c. Allergens, exercise, and irritants are common triggers of asthma attacks. Cold weather, stress, and anxiety are lesser triggers.

51. d. Blood enters the right atrium through the superior and inferior vena cava and is pumped through the tricuspid valve into the right ventricle. From there, it passes through the pulmonic valve into the pulmonary arteries and into the lungs.

52. b. If, on initial assessment, the carotid pulse is palpable but the radial pulse is not, the patient's systolic blood pressure is 60–80 mmHg. (Cerebral blood flow stops below 60 mmHg, so it cannot be lower than that.) When the radial is absent but the femoral is present, the pulse is estimated to be around 70 mmHg. When the radial pulse is present the systolic pressure is considered to be at least 80 mmHg. In light of the complete description given, then, the best approximation of the patient's pulse is 60 mmHg.

53. d. Determining the relationship between the apical impulse and the carotid pulse may give you the first indication of a cardiac irregularity, such as a dysrhythmia. An apical pulse indicates the pump is functioning, and a carotid pulse shows you that the circulating blood volume is reaching target tissues. To assess central and peripheral circulation, you should assess carotid (central) and radial (peripheral) pulses. Remember that the cardiovascular system requires three factors to work effectively: intact and functioning pump, an adequate circulating blood volume, and a container (vascular vessels) of the appropriate size to circulate the blood effectively.

54. b. A second puncture attempt should be made superior to the first because there is a chance of leakage from the first puncture site.

55. c. The history of diarrhea, nausea, and vomiting indicates a strong dehydration situation resulting in the tachycardia and dyspnea.

56. c. Dopamine is the preferred drug for raising blood pressure in patients in cardiogenic shock. Note that it should never be administered if you suspect the reason for low blood pressure is hypovolemia. Once hypovolemia is corrected, dopamine can be administered.

57. b. Apply an occlusive dressing (a gloved hand can be used in the interim until the occlusive dressing is applied), then attempt to stop the bleeding with constant, direct pressure; do not clamp neck vessels.

58. b. The common signs and symptoms of cerebral hemorrhage are transient loss of consciousness, headache, drowsiness, nausea, and vomiting.

59. a. Hypoglycemia may occur in nondiabetic patients, especially in chronic alcoholics who have poor diet and the inability to properly metabolize carbohydrates. Except in cases of alcoholism and prolonged lack of food intake, nondiabetics seldom have problems with hypoglycemia. Signs and symptoms of hypoglycemia have a rapid onset. In early stages of hypoglycemia, the patient may complain of extreme hunger and thirst.

60. d. More than half of all elderly patients who suffer MI do not complain of chest pain; therefore, their AMI often goes unrecognized. In the presence of chronic diseases, such as diabetes, neuropathy prevents them from sensing pain as unaffected individuals would.

61. a. Oxygenated blood flows from the lungs, via the pulmonary veins, into the left atrium. From there, it passes through the mitral (bicuspid) valve into the left ventricle. It passes through the aortic valve then enters into the aorta.

62. b. Since no information is presented about the exact nature of the patient's condition, one assumes that there is a trauma mechanism involved and manual precautions must be taken. A modified jaw thrust can open an airway without disturbing the in-line alignment of the cervical spine.

63. b. Parasympathetic stimulation through the vagus nerve acts to decrease the heart rate; this paradoxically increases stroke volume because the longer time interval between contractions allows the ventricles to fill more efficiently.

64. b. Wheezing localized into one lung only minimizes the likelihood of asthma or other pulmonary disease. If a foreign body is small enough to pass through the glottic opening and carina, it will eventually lodge somewhere in either the main bronchi or the bronchioles. If the obstruction is not complete, air moving past the restricted lung passage will produce a wheeze.

65. d. The P-R interval represents the conduction of the electrical impulse through the atria and AV node, up to the instant of ventricular depolarization.

66. b. Abnormally long or oddly shaped QRS complexes indicate that the impulse was formed within the ventricles and that it then traveled to the AV node. This delay in travel time is shown as a widened QRS complex on the ECG tracing.

67. a. The rhythm identified is a junctional escape rhythm.

68. b. Cardioversion is the recommended treatment for atrial fibrillation when the ventricular rate is greater than 150 and the patient is symptomatic. The other treatments listed are for nonsymptomatic patients or for when you are unclear if the rhythm is SVT or v-tach.

69. b. The most common location of infarct is the inferior wall, characterized by ST segment elevation in leads II, III, and aVF.

70. c. The initial standard defibrillating dosage of energy is 2 joules/kg body weight.

71. d. The standard dose for fluid resuscitation is 20 mL/kg body weight.

72. a. Patients with no respiratory compromise benefit from low-flow oxygen to increase comfort and limit the size of the infarct. Nasal cannula oxygen administration is appropriate provided the pulse oximeter reading remains high (over 95%).

73. d. Any condition that would present a significant bleeding hazard excludes a patient from receiving thrombolytic therapy.

74. a. Patients with dissecting aortic aneurysm describe their pain as extremely severe from the outset, whereas the pain of AMI tends to build slowly.

75. d. Prehospital treatment is limited to elevation and immobilization of the extremity and transportation.

76. c. Delta waves are characteristic of pre-excitation syndromes, of which Wolff-Parkinson-White is the most common.

77. b. Because the patient does not seem to be tolerating the rapid heart rate well, vagal maneuvers should be attempted first, followed by pharmacological therapy if necessary. If the heart rate increases or the patient becomes unstable, synchronized cardioversion may be indicated.

78. a. These features are characteristic of all dysrhythmias that originate in the AV node. The P wave is inverted because of retrograde conduction and is firing virtually simultaneously with the QRS, resulting in a short duration of the P-R interval (if it is present at all).

79. c. This patient is alert enough to be considered stable. However, a heart rate of 260 is difficult for any patient to manage for any period of time. Adenosine is indicated for this condition. Volume replacement is not indicated; there is no information in regard to dehydration or other fluid loss, and a heart rate of 260 may not be able to tolerate large amounts of fluid.

80. b. Straight laryngoscope blades are preferred in children. Uncuffed tubes are typically used in pediatric patients because the narrowest portion of the airway is just below the vocal cords.

81. a. Anxiety is a general feeling of uneasiness or apprehension that results from continued stress.

82. a. The environment she is in and the previously unseen rash, wheezing, difficulty breathing, and negative past history are keys to this being a case of possible anaphylactic shock.

83. c. You should aggressively manage the airway. It may be necessary to carefully intubate this patient, and you may get only one attempt. Once the tube contacts the larynx, the vocal cords can spasm and completely shut off the airway.

84. a. Epinephrine is a potent antihistamine and can reverse many of the effects of histamine overload. This patient is in extremis and should first be treated with epinephrine. If respiratory distress continues once the epinephrine has entered the patient's system, you may try using diphenhydramine (another antihistamine) or albuterol to bring about bronchodilation. Morphine is not indicated in this situation.

85. a. This patient is an unstable patient secondary to supraventricular tachycardia. Synchronized cardioversion is indicated to terminate the dysrhythmia. The standard dose for synchronized cardioversion is 0.5 joules/kg body weight.

86. b. This patient is experiencing heat stroke and possible dehydration. It is important for him to receive fluid, high concentration of oxygen, and active cooling measures to reduce his body temperature.

87. d. Nitrous oxide should not be used with patients with head injury because it can increase intracranial pressure. It should not be used with patients who have pneumothorax because the drug can move by diffusion to air spaces in the body.

88. c. In a stable patient, the PASG is unnecessary. The long board will not adequately immobilize this injury because the muscles of the leg will spasm and shorten the leg. A padded board may not provide adequate traction to prevent muscle spasms either, so the traction splint is the best choice.

89. c. Using the rule of nines, the front of each arm equals 4.5% BSA, and the anterior chest equals 9%; the total burn covers 18% of the BSA.

90. b. The skin over a second-degree burn will most frequently appear mottled red and contain blisters. A first-degree burn will appear bright red and a third-degree burn will be charred or white.

91. c. Severe partial thickness or full thickness burns to the face, hands, feet, and perineum often warrant burn center care, even if they are not extensive.

92. d. Cover the burns with dry sterile dressings and be ready to institute aggressive fluid therapy as needed to maintain hemodynamic stability based on the Parkland formula. Wet dressings offer comfort but lower the body temperature in a severely burned patient. Gel-type dressings are being used with some success across the country in various areas, but the standard of care is still dry sterile dressing.

93. b. Seizures, unlike syncope, do not usually have warning signs such as a period of lightheadedness. Some seizures are preceded by a feeling or sensation of impending seizure called an aura.

94. d. Place the patient in the lateral-recumbent position to prevent aspiration and administer supplemental oxygen as needed; provide privacy and transport.

95. c. Patients who present with altered mental status should be provided high-flow oxygen and IV access; blood glucose levels should be measured. D50 should be administered when hypoglycemia is suspected.

96. d. Injected antigens are likely to cause the most severe reactions; penicillin and insect stings are the two most common causes of severe anaphylaxis.

97. a. This patient presents with symptomatic bradycardia, which would most likely be relieved by increasing the heart rate. Atropine would indirectly increase the heart rate by blocking the parasympathetic nervous system. Epinephrine may be dangerous for this patient due to its cardiotonic side effects and the patient's age.

98. a. This patient presents in a stable, supraventricular rhythm. Because the patient's blood pressure is not low, there is time to establish intravenous access and administer adenosine to control the rate.

99. a. The patient's blood pressure is too low for safe use of furosemide, morphine sulfate, or nitroglycerin.

100. a. This finding is helpful in ruling out acute abdomen as the cause. Acute abdomen generally always has pain associated with rigidity, whereas a spider bite may be painless initially due to the neurotoxicity of the venom. Spiders rarely bite more than once, ruling out choice **d.**

101. a. Tachycardia with wide QRS complex is an important early sign of toxicity. High doses of sodium bicarbonate IV drip will help control dysrhythmias.

102. c. Although any of these individuals could suffer from heat stroke, the elderly person represents the typical profile of a victim of classic heat stroke.

103. d. Alcohol is a CNS depressant. People who do not frequently drink often do so before killing themselves; furthermore, alcoholics are prone to commit suicide. Suicidal patients may or may not openly discuss suicide, but you should take seriously any discussion of it by your patient. Most suicidal patients are depressed, not mentally ill. Holidays and important personal times such as anniversaries, birthdays, or death-days are high times for suicide.

104. a. Unless you know otherwise, always assume a medication bottle was full. There is nothing in this situation to indicate child abuse. Although today the quantity of pills packaged has been reduced, in order to lessen the likelihood of overdose by accidental ingestion, this child's decreasing LOC (level of consciousness) suggests there is a serious overdose situation.

105. c. Salicylates is the correct class of drugs for aspirin.

106. b. The appropriate treatment is IV, oxygen, ECG, and activated charcoal. Be prepared to treat dysrhythmias and to provide a fluid challenge if ordered. Sodium bicarbonate may also be ordered by medical direction, but epinephrine is not indicted for this situation. Naloxone is not indicated in this overdose situation, but could always be given if you are unsure of the substances ingested.

107. a. It is rare to treat PVCs directly; the administration of oxygen and nitrates would be used to reperfuse the myocardial tissue, which in turn may eliminate the PVCs. However, in this case, she is exhibiting more than six per minute, and they are originating from more than one site. Lidocaine may be needed to control these potentially malignant ectopic beats.

108. b. The pediatric dosage is 0.1 mg/kg for a child less than five years of age and 2.0 mg for a child over five years of age.

109. c. This patient presents in pulseless ventricular tachycardia, a lethal rhythm. Immediate defibrillation is indicated to terminate this event.

110. d. Although children are often uncoordinated and subject to frequent falls, the presence of bruises in various stages of healing would lead you to suspect that this child had been injured on more than one occasion. Carefully note the environment in which the child is living and report any suspicions of abuse or neglect to the proper authorities.

111. a. The tearing feeling and the dark-colored blood are classic signs and symptoms of abruptio placenta. Placenta previa often has bleeding that is contained within the uterus due to the placenta blocking the os (opening or mouth) of the uterus.

112. d. Both lives are at stake. Oxygen is passed from the mother to the baby via the placenta. A separation greatly decreases the blood supply to the infant, and the uncontrolled bleeding is dangerous to the mother.

113. a. Administering one or two large-bore IVs of normal saline or Ringer's lactate is appropriate when combined with rapid transport. You should titrate the BP to 100–110 mmHg so as not to overload the circulation, causing pulmonary edema and further compromising the oxygen supply to the infant.

114. a. The most common presentation of PID is diffuse, moderate to severe lower-abdominal pain, which makes ambulation difficult.

115. c. In order to preserve physical evidence of the assault, avoid cleaning wounds and do not allow the victim to bathe or change clothing. If clothing is removed during patient care, it should be placed in a brown paper bag and handed over to police officers. Maintain chain of custody carefully to preserve the evidence.

116. b. This patient presents in unstable supraventricular tachycardia. Her condition may deteriorate quickly; therefore, immediate synchronized cardioversion is indicated.

117. d. Signs and symptoms of ectopic pregnancy include lower-abdominal pain that is often referred to the shoulder, abdominal tenderness, and rapidly developing shock. Although a ruptured appendix may be suspected, the first problem to rule out (given the pregnancy history) is an ectopic pregnancy.

118. c. Placenta previa usually presents as painless bright red bleeding that occurs in the third trimester of pregnancy. The blood may be contained within the uterus.

119. c. Because meconium staining in the amniotic fluid can indicate fetal distress, the best thing to do is transport the mother immediately. Choices **a**, **b**, and **d** suggest that birth is imminent and transport is not advisable. If you must deliver the infant when meconium staining is present, you should be prepared to provide immediate suctioning of the trachea and to intubate the child prior to stimulation, drying, warming, or positioning.

120. a. Suction the infant's mouth and nose immediately after the head is delivered and you can access the mouth and nose. Remember to suction the mouth first, then the nose.

121. d. Immediate defibrillation has been proven to be effective in terminating ventricular fibrillation. Even stopping for CPR in a witnessed event such as this may be more harmful than beneficial.

122. b. Stimulate a neonate by flicking the soles of the feet and rubbing the back. The infant should not be allowed to lose any body heat, and you should avoid touching the head to keep from putting any pressure on the fontanel.

123. b. Increased ICP after blunt force trauma to the head is potentially lethal and will need close monitoring and management both prehospital and within the emergency department.

124. c. This is toxemia, a hypertensive disorder of pregnancy.

125. c. This patient is most likely suffering from preeclampsia.

126. a. Magnesium sulfate is the appropriate medication for the suppression of seizures in a preeclampsia patient. Diazepam may help control seizures, but magnesium suppresses seizures.

127. c. Seizures indicate that the patient's condition has worsened. This condition is called eclampsia.

128. a. Although the online medical control physician is ultimately responsible for the care the patient receives, it would be appropriate to allow the two physicians to communicate while you continue care of the patient per your online direction. You should never leave the patient unless the on-scene physician can be identified to your satisfaction, the on-scene physician has agreed to assume care of the patient, and medical direction has authorized you to discontinue care.

129. d. Bradycardia refers to a heart rate of less than 60 beats per minute.

130. b. Falls kill more elderly Americans annually than any other trauma. It is important to carefully evaluate and manage these patients.

131. a. Most states require the reporting of abuse or neglect of children, spouses, or older adults; rape and sexual assault; gunshot and stab wounds; animal bites; and certain communicable diseases.

132. b. Protective custody is used legally in cases of patients who are under the influence of drugs or alcohol, who are a danger to themselves and others, or when it is obvious that their condition is impairing their judgment.

133. a. Contact medical control about the specific situation before providing care; this will allow you to provide the type of care that is palliative only. Some states have specific protocols to follow with DNR patients and may even provide various levels of care in a variety of circumstances.

134. a. Oxytocin may help control postpartum hemorrhage.

135. b. When using the START triage system, you assess three parameters: respiration, pulse, and mental status (RPM). A patient with no respirations is considered expectant/deceased; if the rate is under 10 or over 30, the patient is immediate. If the rate is between 10 and 30, additional assessment is needed (you would assess pulse, and possibly also mental status, before deciding on a classification).

136. c. Scope of practice is generally defined by state statute and defines what an EMS provider can perform.

137. c. Childbirth can be extremely messy and involve blood, amniotic fluid, urine, and feces, so maximum precautions should be taken to include gloves, gowns, mask, and eye protection. For routine IV starts and IM drug administration, gloves alone should be appropriate BSI. All of the precautions listed are recommended by USFA (United States Fire Administration) guidelines for bleeding control with spurting bleeding but are not necessary with minimal bleeding.

138. a. Hepatitis A is enteric (or food-borne) and poses the least risk for healthcare providers. Hepatitis B virus (HBV) is the major occupational blood-borne pathogen risk for paramedics. Hepatitis C occurs most frequently in IV drug abusers; paramedics are at risk of contracting this disease from accidental needle sticks. Hepatitis D occurs only in individuals who currently have or had HBV infection, and who therefore pose a high risk to EMS providers.

139. c. Treat Mrs. Rodriguez respectfully, and give her plenty of time to respond and plenty of encouragement, before you turn to her grandson for assistance or translation. If it appears that she is nervous about her grandson being present, you may then decide to ask him to leave the room; but, unless his presence is upsetting to the patient, it is okay for him to remain.

140. a. The typical abused elder is generally poor and dependent on the abuser.

141. b. This is one way to acknowledge what a patient is feeling and to encourage him or her to express those feelings without passing judgment or getting too personal.

142. a. Limit your time of exposure, stay a good distance from the source, and place shielding between you and the source. Personal and crew safety is always your first concern.

143. c. Upwind in a building helps to provide further shielding from the radioactive source. Since you will be able to communicate via radio, being able to see the scene of the emergency is not important in this situation.

144. c. Decontamination should only be performed by specially trained hazardous materials personnel.

145. c. Gamma rays are the most serious type of ionizing radiation.

146. d. The rhythm is a third-degree heart block. The P waves are normal and have a regular rhythm, the QRS complexes are narrow, but the QRS complexes and the P waves have no association.

147. b. The ST segment changes in the 12-lead indicate a lateral wall MI. There is ST elevation in leads V5 and V6. The T waves in V1 appear peaked, but the ST segment is not indicative of septal wall involvement.

148. c. The rhythm is atrial fibrillation with a rapid ventricular response. The telltale sign is the irregularity of the RR segment. Since this patient is stable and it is an acute onset of atrial fibrillation, the first-line pharmacological agent is diltiazem at 0.25 mg/kg administered via a slow IV push over two minutes.

149. b. Succinylcholine causes muscle fasciculations (tremors). There is no reversal agent for succinylcholine. Succinylcholine is a depolarizing paralytic that has no amnestic or analgesic properties.

150. c. Hyperventilation will cause an increase in mean intrathoracic pressure, which causes a reduction in cardiac preload. Hyperventilation will reduce PCO_2. Hyperventilation should only be used in cases of brain stem herniation as a temporizing measure to reduce ICP. Routine hyperventilation during cardiac arrest is not recommended.

Scoring

Evaluate how you did on this practice exam by first finding the number of questions you answered correctly. Only the number of correct answers is important—questions you skipped or answered incorrectly do not count against your score. Your goal should be a score greater than 80%. The NREMT exam is now computer adaptive and therefore there is no minimum score, just a measure of competency.

Use your scores in conjunction with the LearningExpress Test Preparation System in Chapter 2 of this book to help devise a study plan. You should plan to spend more time on the topics that you found hardest, and less time on the topics in which you performed well.

Much more important than your overall score, for now, is how you did on each of the topics tested by the exam. You need to diagnose your strengths and weaknesses so that you can concentrate your efforts as you prepare. The question types are mixed in the practice exam, so in order to tell where your strengths and weaknesses lie, you will need to compare your answer sheet with the following table that shows the topic for each question.

PARAMEDIC PRACTICE EXAM 4 DIAGNOSTIC SCORING CHART	
TOPIC	**QUESTION #**
Airway, Respiration, and Ventilation	1, 2, 3, 4, 28, 30, 31, 32, 36, 37, 38, 40, 41, 42, 43, 44, 45, 46, 47, 48, 49, 50, 64, 80, 150
Cardiology and Resuscitation	21, 27, 29, 51, 56, 60, 61, 63, 65, 66, 67, 68, 69, 70, 72, 73, 74, 76, 77, 78, 79, 85, 97, 98, 99, 107, 109, 116, 121, 146, 147, 148
Trauma	7, 8, 9, 10, 12, 13, 14, 15, 26, 28, 33, 53, 54, 88, 89, 90, 91, 92, 115, 116, 117, 119, 123, 131, 132, 139, 142, 144
Medical/Obstetrics/ Gynecology	18, 19, 20, 26, 33, 34, 35, 55, 58, 59, 75, 81, 82, 83, 84, 86, 93, 94, 95, 96, 100, 101, 102, 103, 104, 106, 111, 112, 113, 114, 115, 117, 118, 119, 120, 122, 124, 125, 126, 127, 134
EMS Operations	5, 6, 52, 53, 54, 105, 108, 110, 128, 129, 131, 132, 133, 135, 136, 137, 138, 139, 140, 141, 142, 143, 144, 145, 149

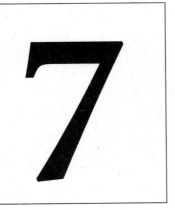

PARAMEDIC PRACTICE EXAM 5

CHAPTER SUMMARY

This is the last of five practice exams in this book based on the Paramedic written exam. Use all of your experience and strategies that you gained from the other four exams, and take this exam to see how far you have come.

Although this is the last practice exam in this book, it is not designed to be any harder than the other four. It is simply another representation of what you might find on the real exam. There should not be anything here to surprise you. Because you have worked hard taking practice tests, you *will* be prepared and you *will not* be surprised.

For this exam, pull together all the tips you have been practicing since the first exam. Give yourself the time and the space to work. Select an unfamiliar location to take the test since you will not be taking the real test in your living room—the public library would be a good choice, as long as your branch is not excessively noisy. You should draw on what you have learned from reading the answer explanations. If you come across a question that you find puzzling, think back to those explanations and see if they can help you zero in on the correct answer.

Most of all, relax. You have worked hard and have every right to be confident!

1.	(a)	(b)	(c)	(d)	51.	(a)	(b)	(c)	(d)	101.	(a)	(b)	(c)	(d)
2.	(a)	(b)	(c)	(d)	52.	(a)	(b)	(c)	(d)	102.	(a)	(b)	(c)	(d)
3.	(a)	(b)	(c)	(d)	53.	(a)	(b)	(c)	(d)	103.	(a)	(b)	(c)	(d)
4.	(a)	(b)	(c)	(d)	54.	(a)	(b)	(c)	(d)	104.	(a)	(b)	(c)	(d)
5.	(a)	(b)	(c)	(d)	55.	(a)	(b)	(c)	(d)	105.	(a)	(b)	(c)	(d)
6.	(a)	(b)	(c)	(d)	56.	(a)	(b)	(c)	(d)	106.	(a)	(b)	(c)	(d)
7.	(a)	(b)	(c)	(d)	57.	(a)	(b)	(c)	(d)	107.	(a)	(b)	(c)	(d)
8.	(a)	(b)	(c)	(d)	58.	(a)	(b)	(c)	(d)	108.	(a)	(b)	(c)	(d)
9.	(a)	(b)	(c)	(d)	59.	(a)	(b)	(c)	(d)	109.	(a)	(b)	(c)	(d)
10.	(a)	(b)	(c)	(d)	60.	(a)	(b)	(c)	(d)	110.	(a)	(b)	(c)	(d)
11.	(a)	(b)	(c)	(d)	61.	(a)	(b)	(c)	(d)	111.	(a)	(b)	(c)	(d)
12.	(a)	(b)	(c)	(d)	62.	(a)	(b)	(c)	(d)	112.	(a)	(b)	(c)	(d)
13.	(a)	(b)	(c)	(d)	63.	(a)	(b)	(c)	(d)	113.	(a)	(b)	(c)	(d)
14.	(a)	(b)	(c)	(d)	64.	(a)	(b)	(c)	(d)	114.	(a)	(b)	(c)	(d)
15.	(a)	(b)	(c)	(d)	65.	(a)	(b)	(c)	(d)	115.	(a)	(b)	(c)	(d)
16.	(a)	(b)	(c)	(d)	66.	(a)	(b)	(c)	(d)	116.	(a)	(b)	(c)	(d)
17.	(a)	(b)	(c)	(d)	67.	(a)	(b)	(c)	(d)	117.	(a)	(b)	(c)	(d)
18.	(a)	(b)	(c)	(d)	68.	(a)	(b)	(c)	(d)	118.	(a)	(b)	(c)	(d)
19.	(a)	(b)	(c)	(d)	69.	(a)	(b)	(c)	(d)	119.	(a)	(b)	(c)	(d)
20.	(a)	(b)	(c)	(d)	70.	(a)	(b)	(c)	(d)	120.	(a)	(b)	(c)	(d)
21.	(a)	(b)	(c)	(d)	71.	(a)	(b)	(c)	(d)	121.	(a)	(b)	(c)	(d)
22.	(a)	(b)	(c)	(d)	72.	(a)	(b)	(c)	(d)	122.	(a)	(b)	(c)	(d)
23.	(a)	(b)	(c)	(d)	73.	(a)	(b)	(c)	(d)	123.	(a)	(b)	(c)	(d)
24.	(a)	(b)	(c)	(d)	74.	(a)	(b)	(c)	(d)	124.	(a)	(b)	(c)	(d)
25.	(a)	(b)	(c)	(d)	75.	(a)	(b)	(c)	(d)	125.	(a)	(b)	(c)	(d)
26.	(a)	(b)	(c)	(d)	76.	(a)	(b)	(c)	(d)	126.	(a)	(b)	(c)	(d)
27.	(a)	(b)	(c)	(d)	77.	(a)	(b)	(c)	(d)	127.	(a)	(b)	(c)	(d)
28.	(a)	(b)	(c)	(d)	78.	(a)	(b)	(c)	(d)	128.	(a)	(b)	(c)	(d)
29.	(a)	(b)	(c)	(d)	79.	(a)	(b)	(c)	(d)	129.	(a)	(b)	(c)	(d)
30.	(a)	(b)	(c)	(d)	80.	(a)	(b)	(c)	(d)	130.	(a)	(b)	(c)	(d)
31.	(a)	(b)	(c)	(d)	81.	(a)	(b)	(c)	(d)	131.	(a)	(b)	(c)	(d)
32.	(a)	(b)	(c)	(d)	82.	(a)	(b)	(c)	(d)	132.	(a)	(b)	(c)	(d)
33.	(a)	(b)	(c)	(d)	83.	(a)	(b)	(c)	(d)	133.	(a)	(b)	(c)	(d)
34.	(a)	(b)	(c)	(d)	84.	(a)	(b)	(c)	(d)	134.	(a)	(b)	(c)	(d)
35.	(a)	(b)	(c)	(d)	85.	(a)	(b)	(c)	(d)	135.	(a)	(b)	(c)	(d)
36.	(a)	(b)	(c)	(d)	86.	(a)	(b)	(c)	(d)	136.	(a)	(b)	(c)	(d)
37.	(a)	(b)	(c)	(d)	87.	(a)	(b)	(c)	(d)	137.	(a)	(b)	(c)	(d)
38.	(a)	(b)	(c)	(d)	88.	(a)	(b)	(c)	(d)	138.	(a)	(b)	(c)	(d)
39.	(a)	(b)	(c)	(d)	89.	(a)	(b)	(c)	(d)	139.	(a)	(b)	(c)	(d)
40.	(a)	(b)	(c)	(d)	90.	(a)	(b)	(c)	(d)	140.	(a)	(b)	(c)	(d)
41.	(a)	(b)	(c)	(d)	91.	(a)	(b)	(c)	(d)	141.	(a)	(b)	(c)	(d)
42.	(a)	(b)	(c)	(d)	92.	(a)	(b)	(c)	(d)	142.	(a)	(b)	(c)	(d)
43.	(a)	(b)	(c)	(d)	93.	(a)	(b)	(c)	(d)	143.	(a)	(b)	(c)	(d)
44.	(a)	(b)	(c)	(d)	94.	(a)	(b)	(c)	(d)	144.	(a)	(b)	(c)	(d)
45.	(a)	(b)	(c)	(d)	95.	(a)	(b)	(c)	(d)	145.	(a)	(b)	(c)	(d)
46.	(a)	(b)	(c)	(d)	96.	(a)	(b)	(c)	(d)	146.	(a)	(b)	(c)	(d)
47.	(a)	(b)	(c)	(d)	97.	(a)	(b)	(c)	(d)	147.	(a)	(b)	(c)	(d)
48.	(a)	(b)	(c)	(d)	98.	(a)	(b)	(c)	(d)	148.	(a)	(b)	(c)	(d)
49.	(a)	(b)	(c)	(d)	99.	(a)	(b)	(c)	(d)	149.	(a)	(b)	(c)	(d)
50.	(a)	(b)	(c)	(d)	100.	(a)	(b)	(c)	(d)	150.	(a)	(b)	(c)	(d)

Paramedic Exam 5

1. What do orthostatic vital sign changes suggest for a patient with acute abdominal pain?
   a. The patient has appendicitis.
   b. The patient is hypovolemic.
   c. The patient has peritonitis.
   d. The patient is a diabetic.

2. Your patient is a 28-year-old diver who has been using scuba equipment. His diving partner states that he was unconscious when he surfaced after a dive. You should suspect which of the following?
   a. type I decompression sickness
   b. type II decompression sickness
   c. air embolism
   d. pneumomediastinum

3. Which statement about the pain that accompanies a myocardial infarction is incorrect?
   a. Patients often describe the pain as crushing.
   b. The pain is not relieved by rest.
   c. The pain is relieved by sublingual nitroglycerin.
   d. Pain due to AMI radiates like anginal pain.

4. You have just intubated your patient with an 8.0 cm endotracheal tube. Which of the following is correct in regard to tube depth?
   a. The tube should be secured at the 8 cm mark.
   b. The tube should be secured at the 16 cm mark.
   c. The tube should be secured at the 24 cm mark.
   d. The tube should be secured at the 32 cm mark.

5. Which of the following is a disease that is associated with cigarette smoking and is related to, but distinct from, emphysema?
   a. chronic bronchitis
   b. congestive heart failure
   c. simple pneumothorax
   d. spontaneous empyema

6. Which of the following statements regarding the treatment of a patient who is suffering from complications of dialysis is correct?
   a. If possible, obtain a blood pressure reading on the arm on which the shunt is located.
   b. Watch for narrow complex tachycardia to develop as the patient becomes hypoxic.
   c. Monitoring for dysrhythmias is frequently unnecessary in a hemodialysis patient.
   d. To prevent exacerbation of the problem, start an IV only if ordered by medical control.

7. A single-lead ECG tracing is useful for obtaining information about the heart. Which of the following can be determined from a single-lead ECG tracing?
   a. mechanical response of ventricles
   b. cardiac output and stroke volume
   c. timing of electrical impulse travel
   d. the presence of a myocardial infarct

8. A QRS complex is considered abnormal if it lasts longer than how many seconds?
   a. 0.04
   b. 0.08
   c. 0.10
   d. 0.12

9. Wolff-Parkinson-White (WPW) syndrome is characterized by which of the following waveform abnormalities?
   a. QRS complex shorter than 0.12 seconds
   b. short P-R interval and long QRS complex
   c. lengthened and bizarre QRS complex
   d. inverted P waves and normal QRS complex

10. What does a prolonged sinus tachycardia accompanying an acute myocardial infarction suggest?
    a. Cardiogenic shock may develop.
    b. Damage to the heart is minimal.
    c. Hypervolemia is the underlying cause.
    d. The diagnosis of MI is incorrect.

11. Which crash has the most kinetic energy and therefore the potential for the most severe injuries?
    a. two-vehicle head-on impact
    b. two-vehicle side impact
    c. single-vehicle frontal impact with a stationary object
    d. two-vehicle rear-end impact

12. What injuries would you suspect in a patient who was an unrestrained driver in a frontal impact collision where the air bags did not deploy and there is deformity of the steering wheel?
    a. compression fracture of the lumbar spine
    b. lacerated kidney
    c. basilar skull fracture
    d. shearing injury of the aorta

13. Which of the following signs and symptoms would you expect to find in a patient with pericardial tamponade?
    a. anxiety, diaphoresis, tachycardia, hypotension, dyspnea, jugular vein distention, and diminished breath sounds unilaterally
    b. altered mental status, bradycardia, hypertension, Battle's sign
    c. anxiety, diaphoresis, tachycardia, hypotension, jugular vein distention, and a narrowing pulse pressure
    d. anxiety, tachycardia, tachypnea, clear and equal breath sounds, and hallucinations

14. A patient involved in a two-vehicle head-on collision has suffered a scalp laceration and is complaining of dyspnea and c-spine pain. You notice that the patient was unrestrained. There is spidering of the windshield and deformity to the steering wheel. This patient's injuries indicate which pathway of injury?
    a. lateral impact
    b. up and over
    c. down and under
    d. ejection

15. An eight-year-old child was riding in the back-seat of a vehicle involved in a frontal impact collision. The child is quiet and the patient exam is unremarkable except for redness and bruising that crosses his abdomen near his navel. The parents indicate the child was restrained by a lap belt. They believe the child is fine and the bruising is from the lap belt. Which of the following is the most appropriate action for the paramedic to take?

   a. Allow the parent to sign a refusal form for the child.

   b. Transport the child without the parent's consent under implied consent.

   c. Advise the parents the child may have retroperitoneal injuries and requires transport to the hospital.

   d. Allow the parents to refuse care and then report them for child abuse.

16. Why is epinephrine used in the care of a cardiac arrest patient?

   a. It increases the diameter of the bronchioles to improve artificial ventilation.

   b. It increases cardiac contractility and dilates coronary vessels to improve blood flow to the vital organs.

   c. It prevents anaphylaxis from lidocaine reactions.

   d. It increases the effects of the other drugs.

17. Sodium nitroprusside is used in the treatment of which of the following?

   a. deep venous thrombosis

   b. myocardial infarction

   c. hypertensive emergency

   d. cardiogenic shock

18. The P wave on an ECG strip reflects what event inside the heart?

   a. atrial depolarization

   b. atrial repolarization

   c. ventricular depolarization

   d. ventricular repolarization

19. What is a primary reason for administering oxygen to a patient with AMI?

   a. to help limit the infarct size

   b. to prevent pulmonary edema

   c. to reduce anxiety and fear

   d. to treat ventricular dysrhythmias

20. What is the normal gestational period?

   a. 50 weeks

   b. 40 weeks

   c. 30 weeks

   d. 20 weeks

21. How should you control bleeding after the normal delivery of an infant?

   a. Pack the vagina with sterile gauze.

   b. Apply direct pressure to the genitalia.

   c. Elevate the pelvis.

   d. Perform fundal massage.

22. A patient presents with symptoms of flushing, itching, hives, difficulty breathing, decreased blood pressure, and dizziness. What should you suspect?

   a. diabetic coma

   b. anaphylaxis

   c. acute appendicitis

   d. stroke

23. Shivering ceases in a hypothermic patient when the body temperature drops below which of the following?

   a. 80°F

   b. 86°F

   c. 90°F

   d. 95°F

24. Which of the following areas of physical examination of an elderly patient is often the most difficult to accurately perform?
   a. examination of the abdomen
   b. auscultation of the lungs
   c. blood pressure measurement
   d. examination of mental status

25. Your patient is a 46-year-old male with a long history of mental illness. He appears depressed and withdrawn. Suddenly, he begins to sob uncontrollably. What should you do?
   a. Administer a sedative to help calm his emotions.
   b. Attempt to calm him by putting your arms around him.
   c. Maintain a quiet, listening, and nonjudgmental attitude.
   d. Motion to your partner to go to the unit and get the restraints.

26. What is the paramedic's primary goal in cases of suspected child abuse?
   a. Gather up any physical evidence to take to the hospital.
   b. Ensure the abuser is arrested upon arrival at the hospital.
   c. Ensure that the child is removed from family custody.
   d. Make sure that the child receives necessary treatment.

27. How should all pediatric patients who have had seizures be treated?
   a. Give diazepam rectally or IV or IM.
   b. Transport to a hospital for evaluation.
   c. Evaluate for signs of abuse or neglect.
   d. Give acetaminophen to correct fever.

28. A patient begins to have a generalized seizure while running a marathon on a hot day. Which of the following procedures should you do first?
   a. Move the patient into the ambulance.
   b. Administer 5 mg of diazepam intravenously.
   c. Establish an airway and ventilate the patient.
   d. Place cold packs around the neck and under the arms.

29. Your patient is a 35-year-old woman who is eight-months pregnant. You note that her blood pressure is 140/90 mmHg and edema is present all over her body. The patient is anxious and complains of seeing spots and having a headache. From this information, what condition should you suspect is present?
   a. gestational diabetes
   b. preeclampsia
   c. eclampsia
   d. hypertensive crisis

30. What is the order of care for a newborn with evidence of meconium staining?
   a. Suction with the bulb syringe; then, remove remaining meconium under direct visualization.
   b. Suction with bulb syringe; then, resuscitate with the bag-valve mask.
   c. Report the presence of meconium to the medical control physician while administering oxygen.
   d. Deep suction the newborn with a nasogastric tube; then, administer high-flow oxygen.

31. Your radio report to the hospital about the patient's medical condition should include which of the following?
   a. the complete medical history
   b. name, age, race, sex, and weight
   c. the chief complaint
   d. estimated time of arrival on the scene

32. Continual reexperiencing of a traumatic event is a characteristic of which of the following?
   a. an anxiety disorder
   b. stress and burnout
   c. cumulative stress reaction
   d. delayed stress reaction/post-traumatic stress disorder

33. How should you adequately ventilate a patient with a partial laryngectomy through a stoma?
   a. Use more pressure to produce adequate chest rise.
   b. Pinch the nose and close the mouth.
   c. Suction the stoma with a soft-tip suction catheter first.
   d. Use a special bag-valve mask designed to ventilate a stoma.

34. What is a major concern when dealing with a patient with organophosphate poisoning?
   a. exposing rescuers to the poison
   b. life-threatening dysrhythmias
   c. explosion or fire hazard
   d. stroke or neurological effects

35. Which of the following medications is commonly used to treat patients who are victims of organophosphate poisoning?
   a. adenosine
   b. atropine sulfate
   c. calcium chloride
   d. flumazenil

36. What is the rhythm in Figure 7.1?
   a. supraventricular tachycardia
   b. sinus tachycardia
   c. atrial fibrillation
   d. junctional escape rhythm

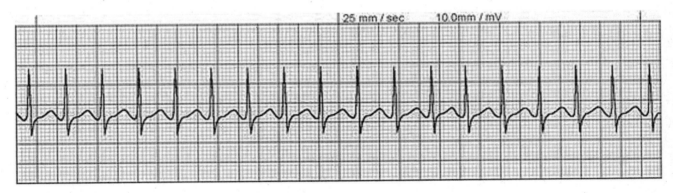

Figure 7.1 Reprinted by permission from Medicine Online.

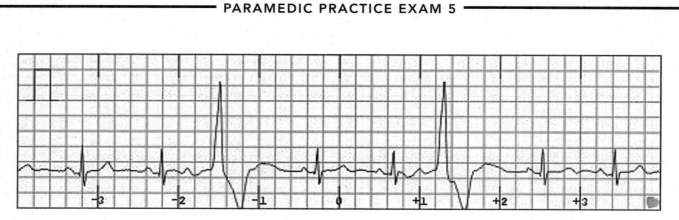

Figure 7.2 Reprinted by permission from Cardionetics.

37. What is the rhythm in Figure 7.2?
   a. sinus rhythm with PJCs
   b. paced rhythm with escape beats
   c. sinus rhythm with trigeminy
   d. sinus rhythm with multifocal PVCs

38. What is the rhythm in Figure 7.3?
   a. ventricular tachycardia
   b. torsades de pointes
   c. PSVT
   d. artifact

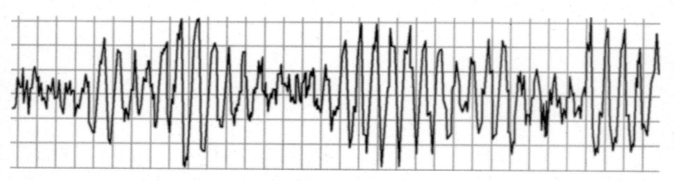

Figure 7.3 Reprinted by permission from Adam Thompson (2010).

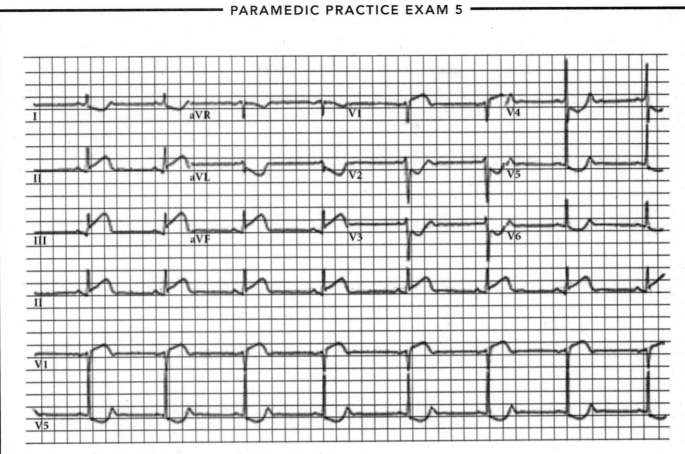

Figure 7.4 Reprinted by permission from Peck (n.d.).

39. You are treating a patient who is complaining of substernal chest pain, nausea, and lightheadedness. Your physical exam reveals diaphoretic skin, pulse of 52 BPM, blood pressure of 130/86 mmHg, and respirations of 18 breaths per minute. You have acquired the 12-lead ECG depicted in Figure 7.4. You have placed the patient on oxygen. What is your next course of action?
   a. to administer 0.4 mg nitroglycerin SL
   b. to administer 4 mg morphine sulfate IV
   c. to assess V_4R to check for a right ventricular MI
   d. to administer 0.5 mg atropine IV

40. A patient in a very early stage of hypoglycemia may complain of which of the following?
   a. drowsiness
   b. dry mouth
   c. nausea
   d. hunger

41. What term best describes a patient who talks nonstop and is restless and overactive?
   a. manic
   b. depressed
   c. demented
   d. schizophrenic

42. Your patient is a 28-year-old female who reports that she is nine weeks pregnant. She is complaining of severe abdominal pain, shoulder pain, and vaginal bleeding. Vital signs are within normal limits, and a physical exam reveals tenderness in the lower-left quadrant. What should you suspect is occurring?
a. uterine rupture
b. ectopic pregnancy
c. spontaneous abortion
d. abruptio placentae

43. What does the presence of meconium on the neonate or in the amniotic fluid indicate?
a. The infant may have been distressed.
b. The infant was born prematurely.
c. The infant will need resuscitation.
d. The infant has congenital anomalies.

44. Your friend experiences severe anxiety when crossing bridges. She refuses to cross any bridges and alters her travel routes accordingly. This is an example of which of the following conditions?
a. psychosis
b. neurosis
c. delirium
d. phobia

45. Where is the location of the infarct in Figure 7.5?
a. lateral wall MI
b. inferior wall MI
c. posterior wall MI
d. septal wall MI

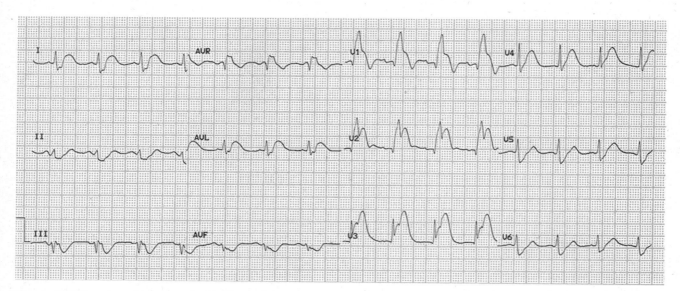

Figure 7.5 Reprinted by permission from Ed Burns.

46. You are treating a hypotensive CHF patient who requires the infusion of 15 mcg/kg/min. of dopamine. You have 800 mg of dopamine mixed in 500 mL of NS. The patient weighs 240 pounds. Using a 60 gtt/mL microdrip administration set, how many drops per minute will you infuse?

　　a. 24 gtt/min.
　　b. 27 gtt/min.
　　c. 61 gtt/min.
　　d. 135 gtt/min.

47. You are treating symptomatic supraventricular tachycardia in an eight-year-old child who weighs 58 pounds. You are going to administer an adenosine 6 mg/2 mL injection. What is the correct initial dosage of adenosine in mL?

　　a. 0.5
　　b. 1
　　c. 2
　　d. 2.5

48. In a motor vehicle crash, which of the following would be most important to understand in relation to the force of collision and the potential for injury?

　　a. speed at time of impact
　　b. weight of the vehicle
　　c. road conditions at the scene
　　d. condition of the vehicle's tires

49. A patient with left shoulder pain may have which of the following?

　　a. bowel obstruction
　　b. pelvic fracture
　　c. pneumothorax
　　d. ruptured spleen

50. Which statement best describes a contrecoup contusion?

　　a. It results from cerebral edema at the site of impact.
　　b. It causes subdural or epidural hematoma formation.
　　c. It is on the opposite side of the head from the impact site.
　　d. It results from open skull fracture and brain bruising.

51. You suspect that a trauma patient has a pelvic injury. She is cool and diaphoretic, with a heart rate of 134 BPM and blood pressure of 100/72 mmHg. Which of the following procedures is most appropriate in the management of her condition?

　　a. two large-bore IVs run wide open
　　b. application of the PASG/MAST
　　c. transport in a position of comfort
　　d. detailed assessment prior to transport

52. What is *ascites*?

　　a. chronic alcoholism
　　b. fluid in the abdomen
　　c. severe abdominal pain
　　d. a ruptured aortic aneurysm

53. What information should the paramedic gather to help predict injuries and for appropriate treatment in a patient who has suffered an electrical burn?
  a. type of electrical burn, amount of current, how often the breaker tripped and reset, and what PPE the patient was wearing
  b. how many phases the electrical service had, what medium was involved in the transmission, and where the electricity entered the body
  c. depth of burn, number of long bone fractures, and the patient's mental status
  d. type of electrical burn, pathway the electricity took, length of exposure, and type of current

54. You are treating a patient who was struck in the chest by a large metal beam at a construction site. The patient is complaining of pain to the left side of his chest and difficulty breathing. Your exam reveals crepitus and deformity over the fourth through eighth ribs in the midclavicular line and on the lateral chest wall. The patient's vital signs are a pulse of 128 BPM and strong; blood pressure of 124/82 mmHg; and respirations of 34 breaths per minute, shallow and labored. The patient has some cyanosis around his lips. What treatment will you provide this patient?
  a. Provide bag-valve mask ventilations, be prepared to intubate, initiate an IV, and transport to a trauma center.
  b. Place the patient on supplemental oxygen at 15 lpm via a nonrebreather mask, initiate an IV, secure the flail segment with a bulky dressing upon exhalation, and transport to a trauma center.
  c. Place the patient on supplemental oxygen at 4 lpm via nasal cannula, secure the flail segment with a bulky dressing upon inhalation, and transport to a trauma center.
  d. Place the patient on supplemental oxygen at 15 lpm via a nonrebreather mask, initiate an IV, secure the flail segment with a bulky dressing upon inhalation, and transport to a trauma center.

55. A patient has fallen while ice skating. The patient complains of pain to her lower back and tailbone. She also complains of pins and needles in her feet. You have completed a neurological exam and found she is unable to push down with her feet and has a loss of sensation on the back of her legs. She has normal sensation on the top of her feet. Which nerve root is most likely affected?
  a. T7
  b. L3
  c. S1
  d. S5

56. What is the name of a brain injury that results in a gradual onset of symptoms; can be classified as acute or chronic; and presents with altering levels of consciousness, focal neurologic signs, and/or slurred speech?
   a. intracerebral hematoma
   b. epidural hematoma
   c. subarachnoid hemorrhage
   d. subdural hematoma

57. Which of the following injuries would require the use of an occlusive dressing?
   a. a laceration to the abdomen with a section of protruding large intestines
   b. a deep laceration to the thigh
   c. avulsion involving the temporal region
   d. amputation proximal to the elbow

58. Which type of hepatitis is spread via the fecal-oral route?
   a. hepatitis A
   b. hepatitis B
   c. hepatitis C
   d. hepatitis D

59. Your patient is a 60-year-old woman who has fallen down her front steps and has possibly fractured her ankle. Which assessment finding may be considered abnormal in this patient?
   a. altered mental status
   b. respirations regular
   c. pulse 68 and regular
   d. blood pressure 128/86 mmHg

60. Which of the following drugs does NOT commonly cause toxicity in elderly patients?
   a. lidocaine
   b. nitroglycerin
   c. digitalis
   d. theophylline

61. Which statement about the vital signs of a patient with an AMI is correct?
   a. Respiratory and pulse rates will be elevated while blood pressure will be depressed.
   b. Vital signs are insignificant because management depends on the underlying heart rhythm.
   c. Vital signs vary greatly since they are related to the area and extent of cardiac damage.
   d. Elevated respiratory and pulse rates are generally associated with a favorable prognosis.

62. Which of the following statements is true regarding prehospital management of a very ill neonate?
   a. Early placement of a tracheal tube is critical in early respiratory distress.
   b. High-flow oxygen carries a risk of oxygen toxicity.
   c. Interventions should be reassessed at 30-second intervals.
   d. Allow the parent to hold the infant during treatment.

63. What is the most common cause of cardiogenic shock?
   a. cervical spinal cord injury
   b. severe allergic reaction
   c. left ventricular failure
   d. internal or external hemorrhage

64. The use of PASG/MAST is indicated for which of the following conditions?
   a. controlling uterine bleeding in a pregnant patient with abruptio placentae
   b. preventing shock in a patient with uncontrollable bleeding in the neck
   c. supporting the respiratory efforts of a patient with severe dyspnea
   d. stabilizing lower-extremity fractures in a hypotensive patient

65. When administering IV fluids to a trauma patient, it is critical to continuously monitor which vital sign?
   a. breath sounds
   b. capillary refill
   c. blood pressure
   d. pupillary response

66. Management of left-side heart failure includes high-flow oxygen, IV of crystalloid solution, ECG monitoring, and the administration of which pharmacological agents?
   a. beta blockers and furosemide
   b. morphine sulfate and nitroglycerin
   c. nifedipine and sodium nitroprusside
   d. labetalol and norepinephrine

67. Which part of the ECG tracing reflects repolarization of the ventricles?
   a. P wave
   b. QRS complex
   c. R wave
   d. T wave

68. Which of the following indicates that an AMI patient is developing cardiogenic shock?
   a. increasing pain
   b. narrowing pulse pressure
   c. falling blood pressure
   d. sinus bradycardia

69. Which of the following is a possible cause of pulseless electrical activity?
   a. right-side heart failure
   b. tachycardia
   c. hypovolemia
   d. hypokalemia

70. Which of these following rhythms might indicate a need for cardioversion?
   a. atrial fibrillation at a rate of 120 BPM
   b. junctional tachycardia at a rate of 120 BPM
   c. wandering atrial pacemaker at a rate of 120 BPM
   d. ventricular tachycardia at a rate of 120 BPM

71. When splinting a limb with a suspected fracture, one caregiver applies the splint while another
   a. holds the limb and monitors distal pulse, motor function, and sensation.
   b. calms, reassures, and provides emotional support to the patient.
   c. checks for limb alignment and administers high-flow oxygen.
   d. gets the stretcher or other supplies and monitors vital signs.

72. Your patient is a four-year-old girl who awoke in the middle of the night with a cough that her mother describes as sounding "like a seal barking." The patient feels more comfortable sitting up. Vital signs are: respirations 26 breaths per minute; pulse 100 BPM; temperature, 101°F. On physical exam, you hear stridor on inspiration. From this scenario, you should suspect which condition?
   a. airway obstruction
   b. croup
   c. epiglottitis
   d. asthma

73. Which situation would constitute a moral dilemma for a paramedic?
  a. a female rape victim who insists on being cared for only by a female paramedic or EMT
  b. a patient who has sustained a potentially serious head injury but refuses care or transport
  c. a patient who signed a do-not-resuscitate order who is now unconscious and dying
  d. a patient who is found unconscious with no family member present to authorize care

74. Which is the meaning of a red tag in the METTAG triage system?
  a. The victim is dead.
  b. The victim has critical injuries.
  c. The victim has minor injuries.
  d. The victim has serious injuries.

75. On reaching the scene of a single motor vehicle accident, you note that the driver is pinned behind the steering wheel. You also note the presence of two sets of spiderweb patterns on the windshield. How should you proceed?
  a. Look for a possible second victim in this accident.
  b. Suspect multiple injuries for this driver.
  c. Assume a high-speed collision has occurred.
  d. Expect that hit-and-run injuries have occurred.

76. A male patient is complaining of crushing chest pressure and shortness of breath. His vital signs include RR 20 breaths per minute, P 54 BPM, and BP 132/74 mmHg. The ECG shows a sinus bradycardia with a first-degree AV block. Which of the following treatments would be most appropriate?
  a. atropine 0.5 mg IV
  b. transcutaneous pacing
  c. nitroglycerin 0.4 mg sL
  d. dopamine 10 mcg/kg/min.

77. Which of the following is NOT a component of the START method?
  a. circulation assessment
  b. respiration assessment
  c. mentation/level of consciousness
  d. neuromuscular function

78. What are the components of the focused history and physical exam?
  a. ABC and LOC assessment and vital signs
  b. SAMPLE history and focused examination
  c. head-to-toe check and treatment of injuries
  d. vital signs and detailed physical exam

79. A 63-year-old male is complaining of substernal chest pain radiating to his left arm and jaw. He is diaphoretic and cool to the touch. The cardiac monitor shows sinus tachycardia. The patient's vital signs are BP 136/70 mmHg, P 118 BPM, and RR 16 breaths per minute. You have administered oxygen and established an IV. Which should you do next?
  a. Defibrillate immediately with 200 joules.
  b. Prepare to administer atropine IV push.
  c. Sedate the patient and then proceed with synchronized countershock at 50 joules.
  d. Administer sublingual nitroglycerin and evaluate the patient's response to the medication.

80. Which are the signs and symptoms of hypertensive crisis?
   a. pitting edema, tachycardia, tachypnea, and venous congestion
   b. paralysis, seizures, and altered level of consciousness
   c. severe respiratory distress, apprehension, cyanosis, and diaphoresis
   d. restlessness, confusion, blurred vision, headache, nausea, and vomiting

81. You should attempt to remove foreign material from a patient's airway with forceps only in which situation?
   a. You do not have access to laryngoscopy equipment.
   b. You have tried, but failed to suction the airway.
   c. You are unable to insert an endotracheal tube.
   d. You are able to visualize the obstruction directly.

82. Which is the appropriate approach of the EMS crew when they are responding to the scene of a hazardous-materials incident?
   a. downhill and downwind
   b. downhill and upwind
   c. uphill and downwind
   d. uphill and upwind

83. The pain caused by myocardial infarction is usually relieved only by the use of which of the following medications?
   a. nitroglycerin
   b. acetaminophen
   c. oxygen
   d. morphine

84. Your patient is a 65-year-old male who is complaining of pain in his abdomen, back, and flanks. His blood pressure is 90/60 mmHg. On examination, you note that the femoral pulses are markedly weaker than the radial pulses. Which should you do next?
   a. Palpate the abdomen gently for a pulsatile mass.
   b. Administer dopamine to increase cardiac output.
   c. Treat for hypovolemia and transport rapidly.
   d. Administer furosemide, morphine, nitroglycerine, and oxygen.

85. Which of the following activities are performed by the paramedic?
   1. maintainence and preparation of emergency-care equipment and supplies
   2. direction and coordination of patient transport by selecting the best methods
   3. priority assignment of emergency treatment
   4. initiation and continuation of emergency treatment
   a. 1, 2
   b. 2, 3
   c. 1, 3, 4
   d. 1, 2, 3, 4

86. Until ruled out by a physician, documented fever in an infant younger than three months old is always considered to result from which of the following?
   a. epilepsy
   b. Reye's syndrome
   c. epiglottitis
   d. meningitis

87. Appropriate management of a child with epiglottitis consists of which of the following?

a. visualization of the airway and insertion of an endotracheal tube

b. administration of racemic epinephrine and nebulized albuterol

c. airway maintenance and administration of humidified oxygen

d. administration of bronchodilators and corticosteroids

88. Which activity is an example of indirect medical control?

a. A licensed physician who does not work in the EMS system assumes control at an accident scene.

b. A paramedic administers nitroglycerin to a patient with chest pain using standing medical orders.

c. A mobile intensive care nurse communicates orders to paramedics while en route to the hospital.

d. An EMS physician tells a paramedic on the radio to administer morphine sulfate to a patient.

89. A person with a serious illness can delegate the right to make medical decisions to someone else by enacting which of the following legal documents?

a. living will

b. durable power of attorney for healthcare

c. do-not-resuscitate order

d. right-to-die order

90. Which statement about the triage operation at a mass-casualty incident is correct?

a. Each patient's triage and initial assessment should take less than 60 seconds.

b. A detailed physical exam of the walking wounded is part of the basic triage operation.

c. Triage assessment of each individual patient takes approximately one to two minutes.

d. Triage personnel at a mass casualty incident should have the highest level of training.

91. Stroke volume can be increased by all EXCEPT which one of the following?

a. increasing venous dilation

b. increasing venous return

c. increasing contractile force

d. decreasing afterload

92. Your patient is a 67-year-old male who smokes cigarettes and has a history of previous MI. He complains of sudden-onset severe pain in his right leg. He also relates numbness and diminished motor function in the right leg. Other assessment findings are diminished pulse, pallor, and lowered skin temperature in the right leg. You should suspect which of the following?

a. femoral artery aneurysm

b. occlusion of the femoral artery

c. deep venous thrombosis

d. hypertensive encephalopathy

93. Which of the following patient presentations would best be managed by a nasal intubation?

a. The patient is unconscious and apneic with a pulse.

b. The patient is unconscious, apneic, and pulseless.

c. The patient is unconscious, is breathing slowly, and has a gag reflex.

d. The patient is responsive to verbal stimuli, is breathing slowly, and has a pulse.

94. Which of the following drugs is administered only by inhalation?
a. albuterol
b. terbutaline sulfate
c. aminophylline
d. epinephrine 1:10,00

95. You are called for a 55-year-old man who suddenly collapsed. He is apneic and pulseless. Initial management of this patient's airway should include which of the following?
a. assisted ventilation with a bag-valve mask at 6–10 L/min.
b. immediate endotracheal intubation and ventilation with a bag-valve mask
c. assisted ventilation with a nonrebreather mask at 10–15 l L/min.
d. insertion of an oropharyngeal airway and ventilation with bag-valve mask

96. Hyperventilation syndrome most often occurs in a patient who is which of the following?
a. anxious and upset
b. asthmatic
c. in shock from trauma
d. a heavy smoker

97. Your patient is an obese 77-year-old woman who has called EMS complaining of a sudden onset of dyspnea, coughing, hemoptysis, and diaphoresis. On examination, you note tachypnea and tachycardia, crackles and localized wheezing, and distended neck veins and varicose veins. You should suspect which of the following?
a. myocardial infarction
b. pulmonary embolism
c. aortic aneurysm
d. status asthmaticus

98. A patient presents with a sudden onset of sharp chest pain and respiratory distress. She has clear lung sounds, a pulse rate of 110 BPM and regular, BP of 112/76 mmHg, and respirations of 28 breaths per minute. Which of the following conditions best describes this patient presentation?
a. psychogenic hyperventilation
b. acute exacerbation of asthma
c. pulmonary embolism
d. pulmonary edema

99. An 18-month-old female presents with lethargy. The parent states that the patient began looking irritable a few hours ago and has become increasingly difficult to arouse. The patient vomited once prior to your arrival. She presents with pale, cool skin; a pulse rate of 200 BPM; and a respiratory rate of 40 breaths per minute. She responds to painful stimuli with a weak cry. The ECG shows a rapid narrow complex tachydysrhythmia.
What is the patient's primary problem?
a. respiratory distress
b. respiratory failure
c. hypovolemia
d. dysrhythmia

100. What are the predisposing factors for the development of hyperosmolar hyperglycemic nonketotic coma (HHNK)?
a. old age, type II diabetes, coexisting cardiac or renal disease, and increased insulin requirements
b. young age, type I diabetes, coexisting cardiac or respiratory disease, and decreased insulin requirements
c. obesity, type II diabetes, viral infections, chronic alcoholism, and poor carbohydrate metabolism
d. coexisting kidney disease, type I diabetes, narcotics use, and noncompliance with insulin regimen

101. On the ECG tracing, dysrhythmias that originate in the SA node share which of the following features in lead II?
a. All P waves are similar in appearance.
b. All QRS complexes are of normal duration.
c. All P-R intervals are shortened and irregular.
d. The rhythm is usually regularly irregular.

102. If it is not treated, left ventricular failure results in which of the following conditions?
a. ischemic heart disease
b. pulmonary edema
c. chronic hypertension
d. cor pulmonale

103. A transmural myocardial infarction is associated with which kinds of changes on the ECG?
a. Q wave changes
b. P-R interval changes
c. T wave changes
d. P wave changes

104. Moving the outstretched forearm so that the anterior surface is facing downward is called which of the following?
a. rotation
b. supination
c. pronation
d. extension

105. A 16-year-old male complains of a fever, sore neck, nausea, vomiting, and headache. During transport, he begins to have a seizure. Which of the following would be your most likely field impression?
a. brain abscess
b. cerebral neoplasm
c. meningitis
d. sepsis

106. Your patient is hypothermic with a body temperature of 93°F. The patient is likely to exhibit which of the following symptoms?
a. severe shivering
b. impaired judgment
c. respiratory depression
d. bradycardia

107. Children of which age group are in the greatest danger from airway obstruction caused by aspirated foreign objects?
a. 1–12 months
b. 1–3 years
c. 3–5 years
d. 6–12 years

108. You must perform chest compressions on a newborn infant if, after oxygenation and ventilation, the heart rate persists at less than which number?
a. 60 BPM
b. 80 BPM
c. 100 BPM
d. 120 BPM

109. What does it mean if a woman is described as *multipara*?
a. She is pregnant and morbidly obese.
b. She has delivered more than one baby.
c. She has never delivered a viable infant.
d. She is over 45 years old and pregnant.

110. Why must your assessment be especially diligent in an intoxicated patient?
a. Alcohol can decrease pain tolerance in the patient.
b. Alcohol can mask signs and symptoms of injury.
c. Alcohol can increase the patient's willingness to cooperate.
d. Alcohol can decrease an injury's effect on the patient's level of consciousness.

111. Which are the blood vessels in the umbilical cord?
a. one artery and one vein
b. two arteries and two veins
c. one artery and two veins
d. two arteries and one vein

112. Which of the following statements regarding febrile seizures is true?
a. Patients suffering from febrile seizures seldom need evaluation at the hospital.
b. Febrile seizures occur in the majority of infants that have a fever.
c. Febrile seizures signify serious brain disorders.
d. Febrile seizures occur because of a rapid rise in temperature.

113. Which of the following situations constitutes abandonment?
a. A paramedic yields control of a patient's care to a physician who has just arrived on the scene.
b. A paramedic yields control of a patient's care to an EMT while the patient still needs ALS-level care.
c. An EMT yields control of a patient's care to a paramedic even though the patient only needs BLS-level care.
d. A patient refuses transport and the paramedic leaves after obtaining a signature on a refusal of treatment form.

114. Which of the following situations is most likely to be declared a major incident?
a. an accident involving a school bus and car with five patients
b. a fire at a chemical plant during working hours
c. a water accident on a state line with two people in the water
d. a fire involving an isolated single-family residence

115. Drawing a patient's blood without her permission may be an example of which of the following?
a. battery
b. slander
c. false imprisonment
d. assault

116. When you are caring for more than one trauma patient at a time, you should change your gloves how often?
a. whenever time permits
b. for each new patient
c. for each new procedure
d. whenever they become soiled

117. You are assessing a patient who was a passenger in a vehicle collision. The patient complains of pain to his right arm and the right side of his chest, and is having difficulty breathing. Your assessment reveals a contusion on his right temporal lobe, a fracture to his right humerus, a flail segment on his right side, and tenderness to the right side of his pelvis. In which type of collision was this patient most likely involved?
a. rollover
b. up and under
c. rear end
d. lateral impact

118. You are treating a patient who was involved in an explosion at a construction site. The patient has several contusions, lacerations, and puncture wounds on his torso and extremities. These wounds are classified as what type of blast injury?
a. primary
b. secondary
c. tertiary
d. quaternary

119. A patient has been involved in an explosion. Which organs would you expect to be injured during the primary blast phase?
  a. solid (liver, spleen, kidneys)
  b. musculoskeletal (skin, bones, muscles)
  c. gas-filled (ear drum, lungs, intestines)
  d. nerves and vessels

120. You respond to the local middle school for traumatic injuries. Upon your arrival, you encounter a 13-year-old female who was working in the science lab when the experiment she was working on exploded. The patient is conscious and alert, and you note thermal burns to her face and hands. These burns occurred during which blast phase?
  a. primary
  b. secondary
  c. tertiary
  d. quaternary

121. A patient has been trapped in a building collapse for 12 hours. The patient is pinned by debris and a large steel I-beam. The technical rescue team is getting ready to lift the I-beam to free the patient. Which treatment should the paramedic insist on initiating prior to the extrication of the patient?
  a. pain management to decrease the stress on the patient's cardiovascular system
  b. IV therapy to help prevent the effects of crush syndrome
  c. splinting of the extremities to decrease the time the patient stays in the hospital
  d. application of a cardiac monitor if dysrhythmias develop

122. You are responding to a motor vehicle versus pedestrian crash. En route, you are advised the pedestrian is a seven-year-old female. Which injuries would you expect to find in this patient?
  a. fractures to the lower extremities, flank, and shoulder, and head injuries
  b. fractures of the lower extremities and back, and head injuries
  c. retroperitoneal, lower back, and upper extremity injuries
  d. abdominal, chest, face, and head injuries

123. Which of the following is the reason why etomidate is administered during rapid sequence intubation?
  a. Etomidate sedates the patient.
  b. Etomidate prevents fasciculations.
  c. Etomidate paralyzes the muscles.
  d. Etomidate provides analgesia to the patient.

124. In a healthy adult, the primary respiratory drive is influenced by the body's attempts to maintain which of the following?
  a. $PaCO_2$ and pH in the blood stream
  b. $PaCO_2$ and pH in the cerebrospinal fluid
  c. PaO_2 and $PaCO_2$ in the cerebrospinal fluid
  d. PaO_2 and the pH in the blood stream

125. Which of the following transport ventilator modes is most frequently used in pediatric patients?
  a. volume support
  b. pressure support
  c. synchronized intermittent mechanical ventilation
  d. high-frequency oscillation

126. During delivery, a loop of umbilical cord presents from the birth canal. You should perform which of the following?
  a. Cover the cord with a moist and sterile dressing.
  b. Have the mother stand to assist in delivery.
  c. Clamp the cord if possible and cut it.
  d. Reinsert the cord into the vaginal opening.

127. Which are the classic symptoms of narcotic overdose?
  a. altered mental status, euphoria, and dilated pupils
  b. excitability, hyperactivity, and hypertension
  c. respiratory depression and constricted pupils
  d. cardiac dysrhythmias and altered mental status

128. Depression is an example of which of the following?
  a. psychiatric illness
  b. psychosis
  c. mood disorder
  d. organic disease

129. You are assisting in a delivery in the field. As the baby's head is delivered, you realize that the umbilical cord is wrapped around the baby's neck. Which is your first step in the management of this problem?
  a. Attempt to slip the cord over the baby's head.
  b. Apply two clamps and cut the cord immediately.
  c. Moisten the cord and transport immediately.
  d. Position the patient as for a prolapsed cord.

130. The primary treatment of metabolic acidosis is to
  a. have the patient rebreathe their own carbon dioxide.
  b. ventilate the patient adequately with oxygen.
  c. administer sodium bicarbonate IV 1.0 mEq/kg.
  d. determine and treat the underlying cause.

131. Which statement about airway obstruction caused by the tongue is FALSE?
  a. The tongue is the most common cause of airway obstruction in an unconscious patient.
  b. Airway blockage does not depend on the position of the patient's head, neck, and jaw.
  c. The esophagus and epiglottis can contribute to airway blockage in an unconscious patient.
  d. The tongue can block the airway only when the patient is recumbent or supine.

132. A dull sound heard during chest percussion may be associated with which condition?
  a. pneumothorax
  b. emphysema
  c. pneumonia
  d. bronchitis

133. Your patient is a six-year-old child who is conscious but not breathing due to an airway obstruction. Which is the first thing you should do for this patient?
  a. Give five back blows followed by five chest thrusts.
  b. Visualize the airway and perform a finger sweep.
  c. Perform subdiaphragmatic abdominal thrusts.
  d. Open the airway with a head-tilt/chin-lift.

134. Asymmetrical movement during respiration typically suggests which condition?
  a. COPD
  b. flail chest
  c. brain damage
  d. hemothorax

135. Which of the following are the signs and symptoms of air embolism?
  a. pruritus, skin pallor and cyanosis, pitting edema in the ankles
  b. sharp chest pain with sudden onset, dyspnea with coughing
  c. dizziness, auditory and vestibular disturbances, headache
  d. fatigue, pain in chest and lower abdomen, nausea, vomiting

136. Your patient is a five-year-old girl who presents with breathing difficulty of rapid onset. She is sitting upright and drooling. Her temperature is 104.6°F. Which should you suspect?
  a. bronchiolitis
  b. asthma
  c. croup
  d. epiglottitis

137. You encounter a patient with a deep laceration to the left side of her neck. The wound is bleeding with dark red blood that is flowing freely. The patient has a patent airway and is breathing adequately. How will you treat this wound?
  a. Direct pressure with a sterile dressing and pressure bandage.
  b. Apply an occlusive dressing and bulky sterile dressing, and wrap the pressure dressing under the patient's arm opposite the injury.
  c. Apply an occlusive dressing and bulky sterile dressing, and apply a pressure dressing around the neck with a twist on the opposite side from the injury
  d. Apply a bulky sterile dressing and wrap the pressure dressing under the patient's arm opposite the injury.

138. You respond to a patient who has been involved in an assault. The patient is alert, anxious, and complaining of severe respiratory distress, and has cyanosis around his lips. Your exam reveals crepitus and deformity to the left side of the patient's rib cage. The patient's vital signs are pulse 132 BPM and weak, respirations 26 breaths per minute shallow and labored, blood pressure 102/74 mmHg, and distended jugular veins. Which is the most likely cause of this patient's signs and symptoms?
  a. tension pneumothorax
  b. ruptured diaphragm
  c. cardiac contusion
  d. lacerated liver

139. You are treating a nine-year-old male patient who has been ejected from a motor vehicle. The patient has suffered multisystem trauma and is showing the signs and symptoms of compensatory shock. The patient weighs 28 kg. What should your initial fluid bolus be?
   a. 280 mL
   b. 560 mL
   c. 620 mL
   d. 1,240 mL

140. You are treating a patient who has been exposed to a corrosive liquid. After ensuring the scene is safe, the patient has a patent airway, adequate breathing, and circulation, which treatment will you provide?
   a. Brush off the chemical, remove the patient's clothing, blow off the remaining chemical with a low-pressure airline, estimate the burn area, cover with dry sterile dressings, and treat pain according to local protocols.
   b. Don appropriate PPE, remove the patient's clothing, flush the patient with copious amounts of cool water for at least ten minutes, estimate the burn area, cover with sterile dressings, and manage pain per local protocol.
   c. Don appropriate PPE, remove the patient's clothing, flush the patient with copious amounts of cool water for at least 30 minutes, estimate the burn area, cover with sterile dressings, manage pain per local protocols, and keep the patient warm.
   d. Don appropriate PPE, remove the patient's clothing, immerse the patient in cold water for ten minutes, estimate the burn area, cover with sterile dressings, and keep the patient cool.

141. You are examining a patient involved in a fall from a ladder. Your crew is holding in-line c-spine immobilization. The patient has a patent airway, and has rapid, shallow, and labored breathing. Your exam has revealed pain and tenderness in the area of the eighth and ninth ribs. The patient has equal rise and fall of the chest, and his breath sounds are diminished on the right side. His vital signs are pulse 132 BPM and weak, blood pressure 96/70 mmHg, respiratory rate 32 breaths per minute, and jugular vein distention. The treatment for this patient is which of the following?
   a. Insert a large-bore catheter with a one-way valve into the intercostal space between the second and third rib at the midclavicular line or in the intercostals space between the fourth and fifth ribs at the midaxillary line.
   b. Apply a bulky dressing to the area of the eighth and ninth ribs and secure upon inhalation.
   c. Insert a large-bore catheter with a one-way valve into the intercostal space between the eighth and ninth ribs at the midaxillary line.
   d. Secure the patient to a long spine board, provide high flow oxygen, and transport to the closest trauma center.

142. After you orally intubate a patient, your partner ventilates the patient with a bag-valve device. You auscultate the lung sounds to confirm placement. No sounds are heard over the epigastrium; breath sounds are present on the right side of chest and are decreased over the left. Which should you do next?
   a. Hyperventilate the patient and prepare for a cricothyrotomy.
   b. Withdraw the tube after deflating the cuff, insert an oropharyngeal airway, and ventilate the patient with a bag-valve device.
   c. Withdraw the tube slightly after deflating the cuff, reinflate the cuff, and reevaluate lung sounds.
   d. Insert a large-diameter needle into the fourth or fifth intercostal space at the midaxillary line.

143. A whistling or musical sound heard on exhalation is referred to as what abnormal breath sound?
   a. snoring
   b. wheezing
   c. stridor
   d. friction rub

144. Your patient is a 51-year-old male with a history of COPD. He states that he has called EMS because he can hardly breathe. On initial assessment, you determine that the patient is in obvious respiratory distress but not hypoxic. You should perform which of the following?
   a. Administer high-flow oxygen and prepare to intubate.
   b. Withhold oxygen to avoid decreasing the hypoxic drive.
   c. Administer oxygen at a rate of 10–15 L/min. via nonrebreather mask.
   d. Administer low-flow oxygen at a rate of 2–6 L/min. via nasal cannula.

145. In a patient with a thermal burn to the airway, it is critical to watch for signs and symptoms of the development of which of the following?
   a. laryngeal edema
   b. shock
   c. respiratory arrest
   d. bronchiolitis

146. You have delivered a child in the field. You have properly positioned, suctioned, warmed, and stimulated the neonate. Your initial assessment reveals the neonate has shallow respirations at a rate of 14 breaths per minute, a brachial pulse rate of 88 BPM, and central cyanosis, and is not actively moving. Which is the proper sequence of care for this patient?
   a. Immediately intubate the patient, initiate an IO line, and administer epinephrine.
   b. Provide blow by oxygen and reevaluate in five minutes.
   c. Assist ventilations with a bag-valve mask.
   d. Begin chest compressions, initiate an IO line, and administer a 10 mL/kg fluid bolus.

147. For which kind of patient is digital intubation method used?
   a. patients who have short anterior cords
   b. patients who are very old or very young
   c. patients who have arthritis in the neck
   d. patients who have suspected spinal injury

148. You can reduce gastric distention during artificial ventilations by
   a. pressing on the stomach during ventilations.
   b. providing ventilations deep enough to cause chest rise only.
   c. positioning the patient at a 15° sideways incline during ventilations.
   d. squeezing the bag-valve mask quickly during ventilations.

149. A patient with hypoglycemia may present with which of the following signs or symptoms?
   a. bizarre behavior
   b. blurred vision
   c. gradual onset
   d. bradycardia

150. A 27-year-old male patient has just been removed from a structure fire. The firefighters bring him to you for treatment. The patient is unresponsive and has rapid and shallow respirations. Your exam findings include singed nasal hairs, soot around his nose and mouth, stridorous respirations, and first- and second-degree burns about his head and shoulders. The patient's vital signs are: pulse 128 BPM, blood pressure 128/88 mmHg, respirations 32 breaths per minute, equal and reactive pupils, and clear and equal breath sounds. This patient is most likely suffering from which level of airway injury?
   a. injury isolated to the oronasopharynx
   b. injury involving the upper airway structures
   c. injury isolated to the nasopharynx
   d. injury involving the lower airway structures

Answers

1. b. A positive tilt test in a patient with acute abdominal pain suggests that the patient is hypovolemic and may have impending shock.

2. c. Air embolism presents as neurological deficit (including unconsciousness) during or after ascent from a dive, or as sharp pain in the chest.

3. c. The pain of MI is not generally relieved by sublingual nitroglycerin, and intravenous morphine or nitroglycerin is usually necessary. It may have all of the same characteristics of angina, making a diagnosis by EMS providers relatively difficult.

4. c. The endotracheal tube should be secured at the 24 cm mark at the lips. The rule of thumb is that the tube diameter multiplied by three equals where the lips should be on the tube.

5. a. In addition to emphysema, chronic bronchitis is associated with cigarette smoking. Either condition can lead to CHF. Cigarette smoking, especially in young and thin males, increases the risk of a spontaneous pneumothorax. Spontaneous empyema is a bacterial infection commonly associated with cirrhosis patients.

6. d. Fluid administration in dialysis patients should be under the direct authority of medical control. To prevent accidental damage to the shunt, BP should never be assessed on the arm with the shunt. Be on the alert for widening QRS complexes due to hyperkalemia. Dysrhythmias are common and, if present, are generally caused by electrolyte imbalances.

7. c. A single-lead ECG, used for routine monitoring, can be used to determine the heart rate, regularity, and the length of time it takes for the impulse to travel through the heart. It tells you nothing about the mechanical response of the heart, of which stroke volume is a part. You need additional lead views to verify the presence of an MI.

8. d. The QRS complex normally lasts 0.04 to 0.12 seconds; anything longer than 0.12 seconds is considered to be abnormal.

9. b. Wolff-Parkinson-White, a pre-excitation syndrome, is characterized by a short P-R interval and lengthened QRS complex. Often, a delta wave is present as well. This condition occurs in three of 1,000 individuals.

10. a. In a patient with acute MI, sinus tachycardia suggests that cardiogenic shock may develop.

11. a. A head-on collision generates a larger amount of kinetic energy, as the sum of the velocities of the two vehicles contributes to the amount of kinetic energy. A vehicle striking a stationery object only converts the velocity of a single vehicle into kinetic energy, and the side-impact or rear-end collision may even reduce the amount of kinetic energy if the second vehicle is moving away from the first vehicle.

12. d. The sudden deceleration caused when the chest wall strikes the steering wheel causes the heart and lungs to move forward at the same velocity the vehicle was traveling before the impact. This movement of the heart may cause the aorta to shear away.

13. c. These are classic signs of a possible pericardial tamponade.

14. b. The patient's injuries and the damage to the interior of the car indicate the patient went up and over the steering wheel and into the windshield.

15. c. Young children who are restrained solely by a lap belt many times suffer kidney injuries that result in severe internal bleeding. The symptoms of a serious injury are usually delayed due to the child's ability to compensate for early blood loss. The alert paramedic will recognize the quiet child with the lap belt injury is at risk for serious injuries and death.

16. b. Epinephrine has alpha-1 and beta-2 effects that constricts peripheral blood vessels and dilates coronary arteries as well as increasing cardiac contractility.

17. c. Sodium nitroprusside is used in the treatment of hypertensive emergency.

18. a. The P wave reflects atrial depolarization at the beginning of the cardiac cycle.

19. a. Oxygen can help limit the size of the infarct by increasing oxygen delivery to the heart muscle.

20. b. Full-term delivery usually occurs within the 40th week of pregnancy.

21. d. Massaging the top of the uterus stimulates it to contract, and promotes control of normal postpartum bleeding.

22. b. Hives, accompanied by difficulty breathing, strongly suggest anaphylaxis.

23. b. Shivering is the body's attempt to regulate body temperature. Shivering continues until the core body temperature reaches about 86°F. Lack of shivering in a hypothermic patient indicates significant hypothermia.

24. d. Assessing the mental status of an elderly patient is often difficult. It is often necessary to enlist the help of family and caregivers to accurately determine if a patient's mental status is different from the norm.

25. c. Allow the patient to express emotion; do not interrupt his expression with questions or comments. It would not be advisable to touch this patient too closely as this may be perceived by him as an invasion of his space or privacy and is not a safe gesture. You should always be on your guard for safety issues when on a scene, but restraints are not necessary in this situation.

26. d. In many states, medical personnel are legally required to report all cases of suspected abuse and neglect, but a paramedic's first responsibility is to ensure that the child is transported to the hospital to receive necessary treatment.

27. b. The cause of seizure activity can be determined only in the hospital.

28. c. While the other procedures are applicable to the treatment of a possible heat stroke victim, securing the airway and ensuring respirations should occur first.

29. b. The patient shows signs and symptoms of preeclampsia (or toxemia of pregnancy) and should be transported to the hospital. The distinction between eclampsia and preeclampsia is the presence of seizures and/or coma.

30. a. Do not resuscitate or stimulate further until the meconium is cleared from the respiratory tree by direct visualization of the cords.

31. c. Although some details of the medical history, such as allergies, surgeries, and medications, are relevant, a detailed history is not. Do not say the patient's name over the radio. Estimated arrival at the hospital is important, but the time of your arrival on the scene is generally not important.

32. d. Delayed stress reaction, or post-traumatic stress disorder, is characterized by reexperiencing of the traumatic event and diminished responsiveness to everyday life, as well as physical and cognitive symptoms.

33. b. A patient with a partial laryngectomy has an ability to exhale through the mouth and nose. Therefore, you will have to close them in order to direct air into the lungs while providing artificial ventilations.

34. a. Exposure to organophosphate is a major concern. Proper isolation procedures are paramount to rescuer safety. According to Environmental Protection Agency guidelines, you must dispose of all patient clothing.

35. b. A large dose of atropine sulfate counteracts cholinergic poisoning from organophosphates and carbamates.

36. a. This ECG reveals supraventricular tachycardia. There are no discernible P waves, the QRS complexes are within 0.04–0.12 seconds, and the rate is too fast to be an accelerated junctional rhythm.

37. c. This ECG reveals a sinus rhythm with trigeminy. A unifocal PVC occurs every third beat.

38. b. This ECG reveals a classic torsades de pointes (twisting of the points).

39. c. This patient's 12-lead indicates an inferior wall MI that is often accompanied by a right ventricular wall MI. In these situations, the addition of lead V_4R will allow the paramedic to identify the right ventricular wall MI. If this is found, it may be necessary to administer a fluid challenge prior to other interventions as these MIs can result in sudden and catastrophic hypotension.

40. d. The earliest manifestations of hypoglycemia are hunger, anxiety, and restlessness.

41. a. A patient who is displaying manic symptoms is restless or extremely active and talkative. The patient may be extremely suspicious or violent. If the patient has bipolar disorder, he or she may swing between periods of mania and depression.

42. b. These are the signs and symptoms of an ectopic pregnancy. Most ectopic pregnancies implant within the fallopian tube and have attained a large enough size around nine weeks to rupture the tube, resulting in intense pain and bleeding. The bleeding from the vagina may or may not be present. Most cases of spontaneous abortion are undetected by the mother, who often does not know she is pregnant, and present as "abnormal menstrual cycles."

43. a. The presence of meconium indicates that the fetus may have been distressed before birth.

44. d. An intense fear of something is called a phobia. A phobia can be disabling; its cause is often unknown.

45. d. The 12-lead indicates a septal wall MI. Note the ST elevation in leads V1, V2, and V3 with reciprocal changes in leads I, II, and aVL.

46. c. Your dopamine is packaged 800 mg/500 mL, which gives you 1600 mcg/mL. Your patient is 240 lbs, which converts to 109 kg. Based on the patient's weight you must administer 1635 mcg/min. This converts to 1.02 mL/min.; multiplying this value by 60 gtt/mL results in 61 gtt/min.

47. b. Your patient's weight converts to 26 kg and the initial dose of adenosine is 0.1 mg/kg. Therefore, 2.6 mg would be administered. Your medication is packaged with 6 mg/2 mL, or 3 mg/mL; you would administer 1 mL.

48. a. Kinetic energy = (mass × velocity)²/2. This means that speed plays a greater role in the force changes during a motor vehicle crash. While the other items are important when evaluating an accident scene, speed has the greatest influence on the potential for damage and injury.

49. d. Bleeding within the abdominal cavity can irritate the abdominal surface of the diaphragm, causing referred pain to the shoulder.

50. c. A contrecoup contusion is an injury to the brain opposite the impact site; it results from the brain's rebounding movement against the skull wall following the initial impact. The coup injury is noted at the site of the actual impact.

51. b. The use of the PASG/MAST as a splint in the stabilization of suspected pelvic fractures is indicated for this patient. Since the systolic blood pressure is greater than 90–100 mmHg, any IV fluid should be restricted to a slow, or keep open, rate. This may reduce any additional bleeding from the dilution of clotting factors.

52. b. Ascites is an accumulation of fluid in the abdomen.

53. d. In evaluating the implications of an electrical injury the paramedic should take into account the following considerations: type of electrical burn (from direct contact or type I, arcing/splash burn or type II, or a thermal burn from ignited clothing or type III); the pathway of the electricity in order to help predict which organs and systems may be impacted; the length of exposure in order to help determine the degree of possible internal injury; and the type of current (alternating current [AC] may trap the patient to the source).

54. a. This patient has a flail segment, is in severe respiratory distress, and is hypoxic. The appropriate treatment is to provide positive pressure ventilations with a bag-valve mask, be prepared to aggressively manage his airway, establish an IV, and transport to a trauma center. Administering passive supplemental oxygen will not be sufficient to reverse this patient's hypoxia and applying bulky dressings to flail segments is no longer recommended. The best splint for a flail segment is positive pressure ventilations.

55. c. The lesion or damage to the spinal column is most likely at the level of S1. Damage or lesion at the level of T7 would be indicated by loss of use of intercostal muscles and abnormal sensation between the umbilicus and nipple line. An inability to extend the knees and abnormal sensation on the medial aspect of the knee would indicate damage or lesion at L3. A loss of bowel and bladder control and abnormal sensation in the perianal area would indicate damage or lesion at S5.

56. d. These are the signs and symptoms of a subdural hematoma. An intracerebral hematoma involves bleeding within the brain; the signs depend on the location of the bleed. An epidural hematoma has a rapid onset and is indicated by an initial loss of consciousness, repossession of consciousness, and then another loss of consciousness. A subarachnoid hemorrhage involves the subarachnoid space; the bleeding mixes with the CSF resulting in blood in the CSF and irritation of the meninges indicated by neck rigidity and severe headache.

57. a. An evisceration calls for the use of an occlusive dressing as does an open chest wound and a wound to the neck.

58. a. Hepatitis A is spread by the fecal-oral route and is most commonly acquired from eating contaminated food. Hepatitis B, C, and D are all blood-borne diseases.

59. a. Altered mental status is an abnormal finding in healthy elderly patients. The pulse rate does decrease somewhat with age but should remain within the normal range of 60–100. Blood pressure often increases with age and respiration rates increase slightly as patients use less of their lung tissues.

60. b. All the other drugs (lidocaine, digitalis, and theophylline) are commonly associated with toxicity in elderly patients.

61. c. Vital signs in MI patients depend on the location and extent of underlying heart damage and the patient's response to the insult.

62. c. Interventions during a neonatal resuscitation should be assessed often, so that changes are noted as soon as they occur. The parents should not hold the infant, although it may be helpful to have them close.

63. c. Cardiogenic shock results most often from left ventricular failure following acute MI.

64. d. Third-trimester pregnancy, impaled objects, and dyspnea are all contraindications for use of the PASG/MAST. In addition, the PASG/MAST is contraindicated with any uncontrolled bleeding occurring above the site of the garment.

65. a. Breath sounds are particularly important to monitor during IV fluid administration because of the danger of fluid overload, which will initially manifest as pulmonary edema.

66. b. These are the accepted agents for pharmacological management of left-side heart failure.

67. d. The T wave reflects repolarization of the ventricles.

68. c. Falling blood pressure, especially a systolic pressure lower than 80 mmHg, together with decreasing level of consciousness, are signs of cardiogenic shock in an AMI patient. Reflex tachycardia may develop as the patient's body attempts to compensate for the shock.

69. c. Pulseless electrical activity may occur secondary to a variety of conditions and carries a grave prognosis. Common causes, as listed in the AHA PEA algorithm, include pulmonary embolus, tension pneumothorax, acidosis, cardiac tamponade, hypovolemia, hypoxia, hypothermia, hyperkalemia, AMI, and drug overdose. Tachycardia is not considered a cause of PEA simply because PEA is a pulseless patient with a rhythm that you would normally expect to find accompanying a pulse. (In other words, tachycardia without a pulse is PEA.) Hypokalemia may cause dysrhythmias, but does not usually cause PEA.

70. d. Based on rhythm alone, ventricular tachycardia is the most likely to require cardioversion. The other rhythms most likely will remain asymptomatic at a heart rate of 120 BPM.

71. a. Immobilization of a suspected fracture is best accomplished with two rescuers. After positioning the limb properly, one EMS provider applies the splint, while the other holds the limb in position and monitors the distal pulse, motor function, and sensory responses.

72. b. These are the signs, symptoms, and assessment findings of croup. The seal-bark cough is a classic presentation.

73. b. This situation constitutes a dilemma because the paramedic would have to choose between the duty to provide care and the duty to obtain consent. If a patient has a signed DNR order, you should honor his or her order. When a patient is unconscious, you treat the patient under the doctrine of implied consent. You should try to accommodate the wishes of the rape victim requesting an all-female crew.

74. b. When using the METTAG system, a red tag indicates a patient with critical injuries who needs rapid transport.

75. a. The windshield spiderweb pattern occurs when a victim's head hits the windshield. Two spiderweb patterns and/or the deployment of both front airbags indicates there is a second victim somewhere on the scene.

76. c. Although his heart rate is slow, the patient is not hypotensive. The other three answer choices address symptomatic bradycardia, not the situation this patient presents.

77. d. Neuromuscular function is not part of the START algorithm. START assesses respirations, pulse, and mental status.

78. b. The focused history and physical exam, undertaken only after immediate threats to life have been corrected, consists of ascertaining the nature of illness or injury, previous history (via SAMPLE), vital signs, and focused exam.

79. d. The patient's heart rate is not fast enough to be the primary source of the chest pain. Therefore, administration of nitroglycerin may resolve the chief complaint, which in turn may slow down the heart rate.

80. d. These are the most common signs and symptoms of hypertensive emergency (restlessness, confusion, blurred vision, headache, nausea, and vomiting).

81. d. To prevent tissue damage, you should attempt to physically remove foreign material only if you can actually see the obstruction with a laryngoscope.

82. d. The rule of thumb when approaching a hazardous-materials situation can be remembered as being *up, up, and away*. This will help minimize the risk of exposure to the crew.

83. d. The pain of myocardial infarction is not relieved by nitroglycerin, acetaminophen, or oxygen; morphine is usually needed.

84. c. The patient is showing signs and symptoms of abdominal aortic aneurysm. Do not palpate the abdomen unnecessarily; treat decreased tissue perfusion and transport.

85. d. All of the activities are related to the practice of the paramedic.

86. d. Fever in a child younger than three months old is considered to be meningitis unless proven otherwise; transport all infants with fever promptly.

87. c. Management of epiglottitis consists of airway maintenance, oxygen, and prompt transport.

88. b. Indirect (or offline) medical control is any EMS activity that involves medical (physician) input either before or after (but not during) the care of the patient (e.g., standing orders, run critiques, quality improvement).

89. b. A durable power of attorney for healthcare delegates the right to make medical decisions to someone else in the event that the patient becomes disabled or incompetent. Choices **a**, **b**, and **c** are all examples of advanced directives, stating one's will regarding medical interventions.

90. a. START and METTAG, systems used at mass-casualty incidents, are designed to be carried out very quickly by minimally trained personnel.

91. a. Preload can be increased by increasing venous return, increasing the contractile force of the heart, or by decreasing afterload.

92. b. The patient is displaying signs and symptoms of acute occlusion of the femoral artery. Aneurysms generally do not occur in the femoral artery. If an aneurysm were present, the signs and symptoms would be different from those presented. Deep vein thrombosis would result in vascular pooling distal to the site of occlusion. Edema would be present or developing in the extremity, but arterial circulation would be unaffected.

93. c. There must be some spontaneous respiratory effort for the blind insertion to have a good chance of successful placement. The presentation in choice **d** can probably be managed by basic airway maneuvers.

94. a. Albuterol (Ventolin) is administered only by inhalation.

95. d. An apneic and pulseless patient is unlikely to have an intact gag reflex, necessitating an OPA to help control the upper airway. A BVM will need at least 10 lpm of oxygen flow in order to adequately oxygenate the patient during ventilations.

96. a. Hyperventilation syndrome, which is characterized by rapid breathing, is most often caused by anxiety; however, it is also associated with many organic diseases.

97. b. This patient displays many of the risk factors for pulmonary embolism; her signs and symptoms also fit. The rapid onset of the problem should lead you to hypothesize acute pulmonary embolism.

98. c. The lack of findings is almost as important as the reported ones. For example, the lack of medical history or wheezes minimizes asthma as a possible cause. Not having pedal edema, crackles, or wheezes in the lung fields, or hypertension reduces the possibility of pulmonary edema.

99. d. The relatively sudden onset of this condition and lack of dehydration history points to a primary dysrhythmia as the underlying cause of her presentation.

100. a. The most significant predisposing factors are old age, type II diabetes, coexisting cardiac or renal disease, and increased insulin requirements.

101. b. In dysrhythmias originating in the SA node, the QRS complex is usually of normal duration because it is still conducting regularly through the AV node. Depending on the type of dysrhythmia, the P waves may or may not be upright and similar, and the P-R interval may or may not be of normal duration.

102. b. Because the left ventricle fails to function as an effective forward pump, left ventricular failure results in pulmonary edema as blood backs up into the pulmonary circulation. Left-sided failure is common following an acute myocardial infarction and can also lead to cardiogenic shock.

103. a. A transmural infarction is also referred to as a Q wave infarction because it is associated with Q wave changes.

104. c. Pronation is rotating the forearm so that the anterior surface is facing down. Supination is the opposite movement. Rotation is the type of movement required to reposition the extremity. Extension occurred when the arm was moved out from the midline of the body.

105. c. While the other answers are possible, based upon the fever, vomiting, and headache complaints, this is most likely meningitis.

106. b. This patient is experiencing early to moderate hypothermia and is likely to manifest impaired judgment, slurred speech, normal blood pressure, and tachycardia. Severe shivering generally peaks around 95°F and continues to decrease in intensity until body temperature reaches the high 80s; it then stops altogether. Respiratory depression and bradycardia occur when the temperature drops into the mid-80s.

107. b. Children between ages one and three who tend to put things into their mouths are in greatest danger of aspiration of foreign objects.

108. b. The threshold for bradycardia in a newborn infant is 80 beats per minute, and the range where you would consider the need for compressions along with other treatments is between 60 and 80 BPM. Any infant with a heart rate less the 60 BPM should immediately receive compressions; but, if the rate remains between 60–80 BPM and is not rapidly increasing despite positive pressure ventilation with 100% oxygen, you should perform chest compressions for 30 seconds, reassess, and repeat as needed.

109. b. A multipara is a woman who has delivered more than one live baby.

110. b. As a mild anesthetic, ethanol can reduce the patient's perception of pain. It will be important to carefully and completely examine the patient for any unnoticed injuries.

111. d. The umbilical cord contains two arteries and one vein; only the umbilical vein is used for vascular access.

112. d. Febrile seizures occur in children because of a rapid rise in temperature and not necessarily the severity of the fever itself.

113. b. Abandonment means that a healthcare worker either terminates treatment inappropriately or turns care over to less qualified personnel.

114. b. This incident has a hazardous-materials component along with the potential to result in numerous patients. All the other incidents may be severe, but should not overwhelm the normal resources for the area.

115. a. In most situations, unpermitted physical contact is a form of battery. Assault is the threat of bodily harm.

116. b. Changing gloves for each new patient contact prevents cross-contamination.

117. d. This patient was most likely the passenger in a vehicle that was involved in a lateral impact collision on the passenger side of the vehicle.

118. b. Lacerations, contusions, and puncture wounds from shrapnel and debris are all injuries categorized as secondary blast injuries.

119. c. Gas-filled organs are commonly damaged during the primary blast phase. These organs are more susceptible to the pressure wave generated by the explosion.

120. d. Quaternary blast injuries are those miscellaneous injuries that may include thermal burns from the explosion or the ignition of materials around the explosion.

121. b. IV therapy as well as other medications ordered by local protocol can combat the effects of crush syndrome, which occurs in patients entrapped for more than four hours.

122. d. This injury pattern would be consistent with the child turning toward the vehicle, while all the other patterns would indicate a person turning away from the vehicle.

123. a. Etomidate (Amidate) is an amnestic that provides patient sedation during rapid sequence intubation. Etomidate has no paralysis or analgesic properties.

124. b. Ventilation in the healthy adult is regulated by central chemoreceptors that monitor the levels of $PaCO_2$ and the pH in the cerebrospinal fluid.

125. b. Pressure support is the frequently used mode for pediatric patients.

126. a. Covering the exposed cord will minimize drying of the cord. Additionally, you should try to insert two fingers into the birth canal and try to keep pressure from the baby's head away from the cord.

127. c. Respiratory depression and constricted pupils (pinpoint pupils) are classic symptoms of narcotic overdose.

128. c. Depression is a mood disorder; depressed patients feel hopeless and helpless, and manifest many physical symptoms.

129. a. First, attempt to slip the cord over the baby's head. If this is impossible, you should clamp the cord in two places, carefully cut the cord between the clamps, and continue with the delivery.

130. b. Treatment of metabolic acidosis consists mainly of adequate ventilation. Rebreathing CO_2 is a treatment for respiratory alkalosis caused by simple hyperventilation. Administration of sodium bicarbonate is rarely needed. Identification of the cause of acidosis is not as critical as identifying if it is present and beginning corrective measures to prevent its worsening.

131. d. Blockage of the airway by the tongue can occur when the patient is in any position.

132. c. A dull sound on chest percussion may be associated with pneumonia, hemothorax, or pulmonary edema.

133. c. The first step in treating a conscious child of this age with a complete airway obstruction is to perform the Heimlich maneuver (i.e., subdiaphragmatic abdominal thrusts). Continue until the obstruction is relieved or the child becomes unconscious.

134. b. Asymmetrical movements during respiration suggest injury to the chest wall.

135. b. All other options list signs and symptoms of decompression sickness; only choice **b** includes signs of air embolism (sharp chest pain with sudden onset, dyspnea with coughing).

136. d. These are the signs and symptoms of epiglottitis.

137. b. These wounds require an occlusive dressing to prevent an air embolism; the bandage must be wrapped under the patient's arm opposite the injury to prevent occlusion of the carotid artery and jugular veins opposite the injury.

138. a. The signs and symptoms are indicative of a tension pneumothorax.

139. b. The initial fluid bolus for a child is 20 mL/kg. The child weighs 62 pounds (which converts to 28 kg) and 28 kg × 20 mL = 560 mL.

140. c. This is the proper management of a patient exposed to a liquid chemical. Wet or dry dressings and pain management vary by local protocol.

141. a. The patient has a tension pneumothorax that must be decompressed. The appropriate sites for a needle decompression are between the second and third rib at the midclavicular line or between the fourth and fifth rib at the midaxillary line. The patient does not have a flail chest and needs needle decompression before transport.

142. c. The original breath sounds indicated that the tube was placed in the trachea, but perhaps too deep. Adjusting the depth of the tube so that the distal end is sitting just above the carina will likely resolve this situation.

143. b. Wheezing, a whistling sound heard on expiration, is generally associated with asthma. Snoring and stridor are upper airway obstructions. Friction rub sounds like rubbing.

144. c. Administer high-flow oxygen to patients with exacerbation of COPD. Do not withhold oxygen from any patient in respiratory distress. Use a pulse oximeter to monitor their SaO_2 levels. If the patient becomes dizzy or sleepy, monitor him closely and encourage him to take normal breaths.

145. a. A burn to the highly vascularized tissue of the airway can lead to laryngeal edema and a blocked airway.

146. c. The treatment of a neonate always begins with positioning, suctioning, warming, and stimulating. Additional treatment depends on your evaluation of the neonate. A neonate with inadequate respiratory effort should receive assistance with a bag-valve mask. If the pulse rate is greater than 80 beats per minute, then continued ventilator assistance is recommended. If the pulse rate drops below 80 with bag-valve mask ventilations, then chest compressions and additional advanced life support should be started.

147. d. Because the digital method does not require hyperextending the patient's neck, it is used for patients with suspected spinal or cervical injury.

148. b. Quickly squeezing a BVM may cause enough pressure to force air into the esophagus. Pressing on the stomach may, in fact, compromise the airway by causing vomiting.

149. a. Changes in behavior are the most common signs of hypoglycemia. Other signs and symptoms include diaphoresis, tachycardia, and headache.

150. b. The signs and symptoms presented indicate damage to all of the upper airway structure, not just the nasopharynx or oropharynx. The patient's breath sounds were clear and equal, which would indicate the lower airway structures were not affected. The structures and the heat transfer capabilities of the vasculature of the upper airway are the most important consideration for the paramedic in the field. Most inhalation burn injuries impact the upper airway and cause significant swelling that may require emergent airway management. It is rare that the lower airway is involved in inhalation burns. When it is, the injury does not manifest immediately and usually does not require emergent airway management.

Scoring

Evaluate how you did on this practice exam by first finding the number of questions you answered correctly. Only the number of correct answers is important—questions you skipped or answered incorrectly don't count against your score. Your goal should be a score greater than 80%. The NREMT exam is now computer adaptive and therefore there is no minimum score, just a measure of competency.

Use your scores in conjunction with the LearningExpress Test Preparation System in Chapter 2 of this book to help devise a study plan. You should plan to spend more time on the topics that correspond to the questions you found the most difficult, and less time on the topics in which you performed well.

Much more important than your overall score, for now, is how you did on each of the topics tested by the exam. You need to diagnose your strengths and weaknesses so that you can concentrate your efforts as you prepare. The question types are mixed in the practice exam, so in order to tell where your strengths and weaknesses lie, you will need to compare your answer sheet with the following table that shows the topic for each question.

PARAMEDIC PRACTICE EXAM 5 DIAGNOSTIC SCORING CHART	
TOPIC	**QUESTION #**
Airway, Respiration, and Ventilation	4, 33, 81, 87, 93, 95, 96, 97, 98, 107, 123, 124, 125, 131, 132, 133, 134, 135, 136, 142, 143, 144, 145, 146, 147, 148
Cardiology and Resuscitation	3, 7, 8, 9, 10, 16, 17, 18, 19, 36, 37, 38, 39, 45, 46, 47, 61, 63, 66, 67, 68, 69, 70, 76, 79, 83, 91, 99, 101, 102, 103, 108
Trauma	11, 12, 13, 14, 15, 48, 49, 50, 51, 53, 54, 55, 56, 57, 59, 65, 71, 75, 117, 118, 119, 120, 121, 122, 137, 138, 139, 140, 141, 150
Medical/Obstetrics/Gynecology	1, 2, 5, 6, 20, 21, 22, 23, 25, 27, 28, 29, 30, 35, 40, 41, 42, 43, 44, 52, 58, 62, 72, 80, 84, 86, 92, 100, 105, 106, 109, 112, 126, 127, 128, 129, 130, 146, 149
EMS Operations	24, 26, 31, 32, 34, 60, 64, 73, 74, 77, 78, 82, 85, 88, 89, 90, 94, 104, 110, 111, 113, 114, 115, 116

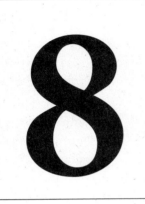

8 ▶ PARAMEDIC PSYCHOMOTOR EXAM

CHAPTER SUMMARY

This chapter is based on materials produced by the National Registry of Emergency Medical Technicians. If your state uses the NREMT psychomotor (practical) exam, this chapter will help you review what makes up this exam. If your state has its own practical exam, you will still learn from this chapter since you are likely to be tested on many of the same skills.

The NREMT has recently made several changes to better prepare paramedic students—not only for the registry psychomotor and cognitive examinations, but also to ensure you are evaluated on how you will actually perform when treating patients in an actual pre-hospital emergency. One of these changes is the requirement that all paramedic students seeking National Registry Certification must attend a paramedic course that is accredited through the Commission on Accreditation of Allied Health Education Programs (CAA-HEP) or holds a Letter of Review from the Committee on Accreditation of Educational Programs for the Emergency Medical Services Profession (CoAEMSP).

A second change impacts all paramedic students: the addition of the Paramedic Psychomotor Competency Portfolio (PPCP), which tracks progress through a student's didactic training from lab work to field internship. All students will need a completed PPCP prior to sitting for the new Psychomotor Exam and the Computer Based Cognitive Exam.

A third change is the psychomotor exam. As of January 2017, the NREMT uses Phase 1 of the new psychomotor examination. In Phase 1, NRP candidates will be tested on five of the current skill stations and one scenario. The integrated out-of-hospital scenario may be an adult, geriatric, or pediatric patient, and you will be given a paramedic partner. The scenario will evaluate not only your ability to manage the patient, but also your ability to manage the call, lead the team, communicate effectively, and maintain professionalism.

All NRP candidates will be required to complete the new psychomotor exam via one of two pathways.

1. NRP candidates who have taken the psychomotor examination prior to January 2017 and are eligible to retest have two options:
   - If you are retesting on either Patient Assessment—Trauma, Dynamic Cardiology, Static Cardiology, Oral Station—Case A, or Oral Station—Case B:
     - You can retest on those stations only as in the past, or
     - You can complete the entire NRP Phase 1 Psychomotor examination and will have two full attempts to pass
   - If you need to retest for either Ventilatory Management—Adult, Ventilatory Management—Supraglottic Device, Intravenous Therapy, Intravenous Medication, Pediatric Intraosseous Infusion, or the Random EMT skills, you must complete the entire NRP Phase 1 Psychomotor exam and will have two attempts to pass
2. NRP candidates who began testing prior to January 2017 and are taking a full retest, or did not start psychomotor testing prior to January 2017, or are refresher or re-entry candidates must complete the NRP Phase 1 Psychomotor examination and will have two full attempts to pass.

About the Psychomotor Exam

The psychomotor examination assesses 5 skills by placing you in lifelike scenarios (via simulated patients and medical equipment) that require you to play the role of the paramedic called to the scene. A sixth station will be an integrated out-of-hospital patient care scenario involving either an adult, pediatric, or geriatric patient. The psychomotor exam process is a formal verification of your hands-on abilities and knowledge, rather than a teaching, coaching, or remedial training session.

In normal circumstances, any equipment needed to complete the exercises will be provided by the testing agency. However, well in advance of your exam, be sure to confirm what equipment is provided and if you need to acquire anything and bring it with you.

In preparing, it will be helpful to look at the NREMT Skill Sheets. These are the scoring sheets that the examiner will use to evaluate your performance on the practical exam. There is a separate sheet for each skill assessed. Check with your paramedic instructors and with the NREMT to secure copies of these sheets. The skill sheets for the 5 legacy skills are available at www.nremt.org/nremt/about/psychomotor_exam_advanced.asp and the skill sheet for the Integrated Out-of-Hospital Scenario can be found at www.nremt.org/nremt/EMTServices/scenarioResources.asp.

A Note about Time

Although the examiner will note the time elapsed for your performance on each section's scoring sheet, the new psychomotor exam has fewer critical failures due to time. The only skill station where your score can be impacted significantly is the Patient Assessment—Trauma station. If you fail to decide on transport within 10 minutes of beginning the scenario, you will fail the entire station. You should familiarize yourself with such time limits and the steps to take for each skill, and practice until completing the procedures in the time allowed.

Psychomotor Exam Content Outline

You must demonstrate an acceptable level of competence in each of the following 5 skills when taking the entire psychomotor examination. The skills scoring sheet breaks each of these skills down into its component parts. You should prepare yourself to know exactly what will be expected of you during the exam by running through these sheets often. In addition, the scoring sheet includes a list of possible critical mistakes at the bottom. Be sure you know the list of possible critical mistakes, as it relates to the minimum standard of care for a patient.

1. Patient Assessment—Trauma

You will be asked to make a physical assessment and voice treatment of a moulaged patient based on a scenario that the testing staff will describe. (A moulaged patient is a person prepared with mock injuries.) This skill entails

- Scene Size-Up
- Initial Assessment/Resuscitation
- Focused History and Physical Exam/Rapid Trauma Assessment
- Detailed Physical Exam

The possible critical failures at the bottom of the scoring sheet include "failure to initiate or call for transport of the trauma patient within the 10 minute time limit."

2. Ventilatory Management—Adult

This and the next part of the psychomotor exam test your ability to deal with cardiac arrhythmias and interpret ECGs. In the Dynamic Cardiology section, you will be expected to handle a cardiac arrest, delivering actual electrical therapy. You will be expected to verbalize how you interpret the scenario with which you are presented and what treatments you provide. This section will resemble a megacode.

The examiner will check 20 steps as you proceed. The critical failures at the bottom of the scoring sheet include such things as "failure to demonstrate acceptable shock sequence."

3. Cardiac Management Skills—Static Cardiology

You will be presented with four prepared ECG tracings, each with patient information. You must say how you interpret each rhythm and what treatments are necessary. For this section, the scoring sheet consists of four boxes, each representing one ECG strip. For each strip, the examiner will write down the diagnosis and the treatment; at the end, as on the other skills, the examiner will note the time elapsed.

4. Oral Station—Case A

5. Oral Station—Case B

In both oral stations, you must manage all aspects of an out-of-hospital call. The sections on the scoring sheet are:

- Scene Management
- Patient Assessment
- Patient Management
- Interpersonal Relations
- Integration (verbal report, field impression, transport decision)

Scoring and Passing the Exam

The psychomotor exam is scored pass/fail, with each skill scored separately. If you pass all 5 skills and the scenario the first time, you have passed the psychomotor exam and are that much closer to becoming certified. During the transition from the 12 skill psychomotor test to the NRP Phase 1 Psychomotor exam, a candidate who has begun the test prior to January 2017 and failed one or more of the following skills may retest up to two times on those skills or may take up to two full attempts at the complete NRP Phase 1 Psychomotor exam:

- Patient Exam—Trauma
- Dynamic Cardiology
- Static Cardiology
- Oral Case—A
- Oral Case—B

A note on retesting for the candidates choosing the above pathway during the transition: Some facilities offer same-day retesting opportunities for candidates who fail five or fewer skills. Not all offer same-day retesting, however, and offering it is not something the NREMT requires of its testing agencies. Furthermore, the candidate is not in a position to pick and choose which skills he or she would like to retest on that or any other day; the candidate is required to schedule retesting on all the failed skills for the same day.

What does this mean for you? Suppose you passed everything but the Patient Assessment—Trauma and Dynamic Cardiology skills the day you take the entire test for the first time. Further, suppose that you really know what to do on a trauma call, and the only reason you failed the practical exam for that skill was a foolish mistake that you know you would not repeat. You might be tempted to retest on Patient Assessment—Trauma on the very same day. However, suppose you also know that your grasp of how to handle a Dynamic Cardiology call is not all it could be, and you failed that skill because you really were not ready to take it. In that case, do not request an immediate retest even though you could pass the Patient Assessment—Trauma section right away, as you would also have

to retest on Dynamic Cardiology. Instead, put off your first retest until you have had time to study and practice Dynamic Cardiology calls.

A candidate who fails any of the other seven skills and is retesting after January 2017 must attempt the NRP Phase 1 Psychomotor exam in its entirety.

If you fail again on both retests (for even one skill or the NRP Phase 1 Psychomotor exam), you will be required to take remedial training for all 5 of the skills and retest on all skills on another date. In order to sign up to take the entire psychomotor exam again, you will have to provide documentation of remedial training signed by the Paramedic Training Program Director or Physician Director of training/operations for your program.

Candidates for paramedic certification who have already passed the NREMT-Intermediate/99 psychomotor exam within the preceding 12 months must follow the same pathways as any other NREMT Paramedic candidate.

Retesting on the Psychomotor Exam

If you pass three or more of the skill stations, then you will be able to retest on only the skill stations you failed up to two times for a total of three attempts. If you fail more than three skill stations, then you have failed your first attempt and must retest on all six skill stations. If you fail a full attempt or any portion of a retest, you will need to provide documentation of remedial training on all skills signed by your Paramedic Training Program Director or Physician Director of training/operations, verifying your completion of remedial training on all six skills.

A Final Note

The paramedic psychomotor exam has just one purpose—to ensure that practicing paramedics are ready to provide quality emergency medical care in a compassionate and efficient manner to patients in the field. The examiners will do everything possible to make sure that the standards of competency are sufficiently high. They will also make every effort to ensure that the test is clear and fair. The equipment you need will be provided; there will be no equipment irrelevant to the situation. No one is going to throw you a curve ball. It is your responsibility to prepare ahead of time by:

- becoming very well acquainted with the steps that you are expected to carry out on each skill
- practicing both the oral stations and psychomotor skills with other students
- knowing, by heart, what would count as a critical failure on any skill

If you do your part, the examiners will know it and you will pass with flying colors. Good luck!

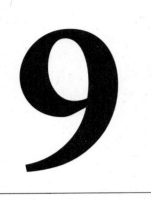

9 ▶ STATE CERTIFICATION REQUIREMENTS

CHAPTER SUMMARY
This chapter outlines paramedic certification requirements for all 50 states and the District of Columbia. It also lists state EMT agencies you can contact for more information about certification requirements.

Table 9.1 identifies some of the minimum requirements necessary to become certified as a paramedic in all 50 states and the District of Columbia. A complete listing of all state certifying agencies is also provided along with contact information. Some minimum requirements are fairly standard and, therefore, not listed in the table. For example, one must be physically, mentally, and emotionally able to perform all the tasks of a paramedic. It is also necessary to have a high school diploma or GED prior to attending training, as is a clean criminal record. Finally, successful completion of an approved paramedic training program that meets the standards set forth by the U.S. Department of Transportation as well as current ACLS certification are required for sitting for state certification and NREMT certification exams.

From time to time, states will change the requirements for paramedic certification. To obtain the most accurate information for each state, you must contact that state's EMS Office. The information provided in this chapter is current as of the time of writing, but does not guarantee that the information will remain unchanged.

The second column of the table, Time to Become Certified, means the amount of time one has between completion of an approved paramedic training program and successfully meeting the certification requirements. If too much time passes between taking the course and passing the exam, one might end up having to take the entire paramedic training program again! In some states, the exam comes immediately following training. If this is the case, *immediate* is listed in this column.

States either use their own written and practical skills exams, exams from the NREMT, or a combination of both. The entry under the Exam column will be *state*, meaning the state has its own exam, *NREMT* for National Registry of Emergency Medical Technicians, or something indicating a combination of both exams. Even when the state has its own exam, it will be similar to the NREMT exam and, therefore, to the exams in this book. The federal government mandates the education standards of the paramedic courses nationwide, so exams are usually similar and based on the National Highway Traffic Safety Administration's Emergency Medical Services Education Standards for paramedics as well as the most current guidelines for American Heart Association Advanced Cardiac Life Support (ACLS).

Each state has its own rules and regulations surrounding certification. Some states have residency requirements for certification/reciprocity. Some states require NREMT certification for initial state certification/ licensure, but do not require the paramedic to maintain NREMT certification. Texas and Oregon require that paramedics possess a minimum of an associate's degree in paramedicine or a bachelor's degree in any subject prior to achieving licensure. If you are unaware of the requirements for your state, it is strongly recommended that you thoroughly research such requirements prior to completing your initial paramedic training. Better to know all the requirements up front, as responsibility rests solely with you, the applicant.

Some states have been looking at moving away from NREMT certification as a requirement in favor of administering their own cognitive exam due to complaints over the new CAT system used by the NREMT. The percentage of candidates "showing competency" (i.e., pass rates) on the first attempt have been reduced significantly since the CAT system was introduced in 2007. NREMT insists, however, that the testing system is accurate and ensures a higher level of confidence that those who pass the CAT examination will be competent paramedics.

The fourth column in Table 9.1 lists whether a state with its own certification exam also accepts the NREMT exam. Under Accepts National Registry, the possible entries are *no*, meaning the state requires successful completion of their own certification process; *yes*, meaning that you can be certified in the state if you are already certified by the NREMT; or *with state*, meaning that if you are certified by the NREMT, you can be certified in the state by taking the state's written and practical skills exams. If the entry under Exam in the previous column is *NREMT*, then that state accepts the NREMT exam.

The same idea follows under the Accepts Out-of-State Certification column; the state will either not accept certification from another state (reciprocity), does accept it, or accepts it only if you successfully complete their certification exams as well. Some states require that you be certified through NREMT if you are transferring in from another state. For these states, the entry will be *With NREMT*. In most cases, a state that accepts out-of-state certification will insist that the training program and certification exams meet or exceed its own standards, so whether or not a state accepts your credentials for reciprocity may be made on an individual basis.

Some states also have additional certification requirements for transferring paramedics, such as background investigations, state residency requirements, employment with an EMS agency in that state, or mandatory refresher training. If you are certified in another state, you will need to show proof of current certification when applying for reciprocity.

Some states have what is known as legal recognition, which means they will recognize and accept your training for a limited time period, often one year. This is similar to a temporary certification. During this period, you must apply for official certification and fulfill all necessary requirements. Once this process is complete, your certification will be good for the normal certification period. Check with the appropriate state EMS-certification agency office for further details.

The Recertification column indicates the number of years a certification remains valid prior to the need to recertify. Recertification usually requires a given number of hours of continuing education, demonstration of continuing ability to perform necessary skills, or both. Again, check with the certifying agency in the state you will be employed for further information on recertification requirements.

	TABLE 9.1 STATE CERTIFICATION REQUIREMENTS				
STATE	TIME TO BECOME CERTIFIED	EXAM	ACCEPTS NATIONAL REGISTRY	ACCEPTS OUT-OF-STATE CERTIFICATION	RECERTIFICATION
Alabama	2 years	NREMT	Yes	With NREMT	1 or 2 years
Alaska	2 years	NREMT	Yes	With NREMT	2 years
Arizona	2 years	NREMT	Yes	With NREMT and state refresher course	2 years
Arkansas	1 year	NREMT	Yes	With NREMT and state exams	2 years
California	2 years	NREMT	Yes	With NREMT	2 years
Colorado	2 years	NREMT	Yes	NREMT	3 years
Connecticut	Immediate	NREMT	Yes	With NREMT or some states by endorsement	1 year
Delaware	2 years	NREMT	Yes	With NREMT and certification process	2 years
District of Columbia	Immediate	NREMT	Yes	With NREMT	2 years
Florida	2 years	NREMT	Yes	With NREMT	2 years
Georgia	2 years	NREMT	Yes	With NREMT	2 years
Hawaii	2 years	NREMT	Yes, with proof of equivalent education	With NREMT and proof of equivalent education	2 years
Idaho	2 years	NREMT	Yes	With NREMT, equivalent education or state transition course, Extrication Awareness, and landing zone (LZ) course	2 years
Illinois	1 year	NREMT or state	Yes	Yes	4 years
Indiana	1 year	NREMT	Yes	With NREMT and state exam	2 years
Iowa	1 year	NREMT	Yes	With NREMT	2 years
Kansas	1 year	NREMT	Yes	Yes	2 years
Kentucky	2 years	NREMT	Yes	With NREMT and determination of death and HIV/AIDS course	2 years
Louisiana	2 years	NREMT	Yes	With NREMT	2 years
Maine	1 year	NREMT	Yes	Yes	3 years
Maryland	Immediate	NREMT and state	With state	With NREMT and state ALS protocol exam	2 years
Massachusetts	2 years	NREMT	Yes	With NREMT	2 years
Michigan	2 years	NREMT	Yes	With NREMT	3 years

STATE	TIME TO BECOME CERTIFIED	EXAM	ACCEPTS NATIONAL REGISTRY	ACCEPTS OUT-OF-STATE CERTIFICATION	RECERTIFICATION
Minnesota	2 years	NREMT	Yes	With NREMT	2 years
Mississippi	2 years	NREMT	Yes	With NREMT	2 years
Missouri	3 years	NREMT	Yes	With NREMT	5 years
Montana	2 years	NREMT	Yes	With NREMT	2 years
Nebraska	2 years	NREMT	Yes	With NREMT	2 years
Nevada	2 years	NREMT	Yes	With NREMT	2 years
New Hampshire	2 years	NREMT	Yes	With NREMT	2 years
New Jersey	1 year	NREMT	Yes	With NREMT	2 years
New Mexico	2 years	NREMT	Yes	With NREMT	2 years
New York	1 year	NREMT if passed in last 18 months and state	Yes	Yes, with NY state exam/ determined on a case-by-case basis	3 years
North Carolina	1 year	State	Yes	Yes	4 years
North Dakota	2 years	NREMT	Yes	With NREMT	2 years
Ohio	2 years	NREMT	Yes	With NREMT	3 years
Oklahoma	2 years	NREMT	Yes	With NREMT	2 years
Oregon	2 years	NREMT	Yes	With NREMT	2 years
Pennsylvania	2 years	NREMT	Yes	Yes	2 years
Rhode Island	3 years	NREMT	Yes	With NREMT	2 years
South Carolina	2 years	NREMT	Yes	With NREMT	3 years
South Dakota	2 years	NREMT	Yes	With NREMT	2 years
Tennessee	2 year	State , with state exam	Yes	Yes, with state exam	2 years
Texas	2 years	NREMT	Yes	With NREMT	4 years
Utah	4 months	NREMT	Yes	NREMT and state skills exam	4 years
Vermont	2 years	NREMT	Yes	With NREMT	2 years
Virginia	2 years	NREMT	Yes	With NREMT	3 years
Washington	1 year	NREMT	Yes	NREMT	3 years
West Virginia	2 years	NREMT	Yes	Yes, with WV legal recognition exam	2 years
Wisconsin	2 years	NREMT	Yes	With NREMT	2 years
Wyoming	2 years	NREMT and state	Yes	Yes	2 years

**Although many states offer reciprocity for NREMT or State certifications, there are limitations. All reciprocity is based on the Paramedic providing proof of equivalent training. If they cannot provide documentation of equivalent training, then the state may not offer reciprocity or require them to take the NREMT or a state exam.

Some states have paramedic certifications; others have licensure. Most states require legal recognition/licensure in addition to NREMT certification in order to legally function as a paramedic. Texas requires all paramedics seeking licensure to have a two-year college degree in the EMS field or a four-year degree in any field. Oregon requires paramedics obtaining licensure to possess an associate's degree in paramedicine or the equivalent.

State EMT Agencies

The following is a list of the agencies that control EMT certification in each state, along with mailing addresses, phone numbers, and websites. Contact these organizations for additional information about specific certification requirements. You can also visit the LearningExpress EMS website for links and additional information at www.learnatest.com.

Alabama
Alabama Department of Public Health Office of
    EMS and Trauma
The RSA Tower
201 Monroe Street, Suite 1100
Montgomery, AL 36104
Telephone: 334-206-5383
Fax: 334-206-0364
Website: www.adph.org/ems/

Alaska
Emergency Medical Services Unit
Division of Public Health
410 Willoughby Ave, Room 110
Juneau, AK 99811-0616
Telephone: 907-465-3027
Fax: 907-465-8741
Website: http://dhss.alaska.gov/dph/Emergency/
    Pages/ems/default.aspx

Arizona
Arizona Department of Health Services Bureau of
    Emergency Medical Services and Trauma System
150 N. 18th Avenue, Suite 540
Phoenix, AZ 85007
Telephone: 602-364-3150
Toll-Free Telephone: 1-800-200-8523
Fax: 602-364-3568
Website: http://www.azdhs.gov/preparedness/
    emergency-medical-services-trauma-system/
    index.php

Arkansas
Division of Emergency Medical Services and
    Trauma Systems
Arkansas Department of Health
5800 West 10th Street, Suite 800
Little Rock, AR 72204
Telephone: 501-661-2262
Website: www.healthyarkansas.com/ems

California
Emergency Medical Services Authority
10901 Gold Center Drive, Suite 400
Rancho Cordova, CA 95670-6073
Telephone: 916-323-9875
Fax: 916-324-2875
Website: https://www.colorado.gov/pacific/cdphe/
    categories/services-and-information/health/
    emergency-care

Colorado
Colorado Department of Public Health & Environ-
    ment, EMS Division
4300 Cherry Creek Drive South
Denver, CO 80246-1530
Telephone: 303-692-2980
Fax: 303-691-7720
E-mail: cdphe.emtcert@state.co.us
Website: http://www.colorado.gov/cs/Satellite/
    CDPHE-EM/CBON/1251589439749

Connecticut
Connecticut Department of Public Health
Office of Emergency Medical Services
410 Capitol Avenue MS # 12 EMS
P.O. Box 340308
Hartford, CT 06134-0308
Telephone: 860-509-7975
Fax: 860-920-3142
Website: www.ct.gov/dph/cwp/view.asp?a=3127&
    q=387362&dphNav_GID=1827&dphNav_
    GID=1827

Delaware

Division of Public Health, Department of Health and
  Social Services
Office of EMS
Blue Hen Corporate Center
417 Federal Street
Jesse Cooper Building
Dover, DE 19901
Telephone: 302-223-1350
Fax: 302-223-1330
Website: http://www.dhss.delaware.gov/dph/ems/
  ems.html

District of Columbia

Government of the District of Columbia Department
  of Health
Emergency Medical Services Division of the Depart-
  ment of Health
899 North Capital Street NE
Washington, DC 20002
Telephone: 202-671-4222
Fax: 202-671-0707
Website: doh.dc.gov/service/emergency-medical
  -services

Florida

Bureau of Emergency Medical Services
Florida Department of Health
4052 Bald Cypress Way, Bin C85
Tallahassee, FL 32399-3285
Telephone: 850-488-0595
Fax: 850-921-6365
Website: http://www.floridahealth.gov/licensing-
  and-regulation/emt-paramedics/contact-info.html

Georgia

Office of EMS/Trauma
2600 Skyland Drive NE, Lower Level
Brookhaven, GA 30319
Telephone: 404-679-0547
Fax: 404-679-0526
Website: https://dph.georgia.gov/EMS

Hawaii

State of Hawaii Department of Health
Emergency Medical Services and Injury Prevention
  System Branch
3675 Kilauea Avenue
Trotter Building, Basement Level
Honolulu, HI 96816
Telephone: 808-733-9210
Fax: 808-733-9216
Website: http://health.hawaii.gov/ems/

Idaho

Idaho EMS Bureau
2224 E. Old Penitentiary Rd
Boise, ID 83712
Telephone: 877-554-3367
Fax: 208-334-4015
E-mail: EMSPROVLIC@dhw.idaho.gov
Website: http://healthandwelfare.idaho.gov/
  medical/emergencymedicalservices/tabid/117/
  default.asp

Illinois

Illinois Department of Public Health
Division of EMS and Highway Safety
422 South Fifth Street, Floor 3
Springfield, IL 62701
Telephone: 217-785-2080
Fax: 217-557-3481
E-mail: DPH.EMTLIC@illinois.gov
Website: http://www.dph.illinois.gov/topics
  -services/emergency-preparedness-response/ems

Indiana

Indiana Department of Homeland Security
EMS Certifications, E239, IGC-S
302 W. Washington St.
Indianapolis, IN 46204-2739
Telephone: 317-232-6425
Toll-Free Telephone: 800-666-7784
Fax: 317-233-0497
Website: www.in.gov/dhs/3525.htm

Iowa

Iowa Department of Public Health
Bureau of EMS
Lucas State Office Building
321 E. 12th Street
Des Moines, IA 50319
Telephone: 1-800-728-3367
Fax: 515-281-0488
Website: http://idph.iowa.gov/bets/ems

Kansas

Kansas Board of Emergency Medical Services
Landon State Office Building
900 SW Jackson Street, Suite 1031
Topeka, KS 66612-1228
Telephone: 785-296-7296
Fax: 785-296-6212
Website: www.ksbems.org/

Kentucky

Kentucky Board of Emergency Medical Services
118 James Court, Suite 50
Lexington, KY 40505
Telephone: 859-256-3565
Toll-Free Telephone: 1-866-97KBEMS
Fax: 859-256-3128
Website: www.kbems.kctcs.edu/

Louisiana

Louisiana DHH /OPH, Bureau of EMS
628 N. 4th Street
3rd Floor
Baton Rouge, LA 70802
Telephone: 844-452-2367
Fax: 225-925-3832
Website: http://www.dhh.state.la.us/index.cfm/
subhome/28

Maine

Maine Emergency Medical Services
Department of Public Safety
45 Commerce Drive, Suite 1
152 State House Station
Augusta, ME 04333-0152
Telephone: 207-626-3860
Fax: 207-287-6251
Website: http://www.maine.gov/ems/

Maryland

Maryland Institute for EMS Services
653 W. Pratt Street
Baltimore, MD 21201-1536
Telephone: 410-706-3666
Toll-Free Telephone: 800-762-7157
Fax: 410-706-2367
Website: www.miemss.umaryland.edu/

Massachusetts

Office of Emergency Medical Services
99 Chauncy Street, 11th Floor
Boston, MA 02111
Telephone: 617-753-7300
Fax: 617-753-7320
Website: www.mass.gov/dph/oems

Michigan

Michigan Department of Health & Human Services
(MDHHS)
Bureau of EMS, Trauma, & Preparedness (BETP)
Division of EMS and Trauma
P.O. Box 30207
Lansing, MI 48909-0207
Telephone: 517-241-0179
Fax: 517-335-9434
Website: www.michigan.gov/ems

Minnesota

Minnesota EMS Regulatory Board
2829 University Avenue SE, Suite 310
Minneapolis, MN 55414-3250
Telephone: 651-201-2800
Fax: 651-201-2812
Website: www.emsrb.state.mn.us

Mississippi

Mississippi Department of Health
EMS/Trauma Care System
P.O. Box 1700
570 East Woodrow Wilson, Annex 309
Jackson, MS 39215-1700
Telephone: 601-576-7380
Fax: 601-576-7373
Website: www.ems.ms.gov

Missouri

Bureau of Emergency Medical Services
Missouri Department of Health and Senior Services
P.O. Box 570
Jefferson City, MO 65102-0570
Telephone: 573-751-6356
Fax: 573-751-6348
Website: health.mo.gov/safety/ems/index.php

Montana

EMS and Trauma Systems Section
Montana Department of Public Health and Human
    Services
1400 Broadway, Room C314
PO Box 202951
Helena, MT 59620
Fax: 406-444-3895
Website: http://dphhs.mt.gov/publichealth/emsts

Nebraska

Nebraska Department of Health and Human
    Services—Regulation and Licensure
Licensing and Regulatory Affairs
P.O. Box 94986
Lincoln, NE 68509-4986
Telephone: 402-471-2299
Toll-Free Telephone: 800-422-3460
Fax: 402-742-1152
Website: http://dhhs.ne.gov/publichealth/
    nebraskaems/pages/home.aspx

Nevada

Nevada Emergency Medical Services
4150 Technology Way, Suite 101
Carson City, NV 89706
Telephone: 775-687-7590
Fax: 775-687-7595
Website: http://dpbh.nv.gov/Reg/EMS/EMS-home/

New Hampshire

New Hampshire Department of Safety
Division of Fire Standards and Training and Emer-
    gency Medical Services
Bureau of Emergency Medical Services
Richard M. Flynn Fire Academy
33 Hazen Drive
Concord, NH 03305
Telephone: 603-223-4200
Toll-Free Telephone: 888-827-5367
Fax: 603-271-4567
Website: www.nh.gov/safety/divisions/fstems/ems

New Jersey

New Jersey Department of Health and Senior Ser-
    vices
Office of Emergency Medical Services
P.O. Box 360
Trenton, NJ 08625-0360
Telephone: 609-633-7777
Fax: 609-633-7954
Website: www.state.nj.us/health/ems/

New Mexico

New Mexico EMS Bureau
1301 Siler Road, Building F
Santa Fe, NM 87502
Telephone: 505-476-8200
Fax: 505-471-2122
Website: www.nmems.org/

New York

New York State Department of Health
Bureau of Emergency Medical Services
Central Office
875 Central Avenue
Albany, NY 12206-1388
Telephone: 518-402-0996
Fax: 518-402-0985
Website: www.health.state.ny.us/nysdoh/ems
    /main.htm

North Carolina
North Carolina Division of Health Service Regulation
Office of Emergency Medical Services
2707 Mail Service Center
Raleigh, NC 27699-2707
Telephone: 919-855-3935
Fax: 919-733-7021
Website: www.ncdhhs.gov/dhsr/EMS/ems.htm

North Dakota
North Dakota Department of Health
Division of Emergency Medical Systems
1720 Burlington Dr
Bismarck, ND 58504
Telephone: 701-328-2270
Fax: 701-328-0357
Website: www.health.nd.gov/epr/emergency
   -medical-systems/

Ohio
Ohio Department of Public Safety
Emergency Medical Services
1970 West Broad Street
Columbus, OH 43218-2073
Telephone: 614-466-9447
Toll-Free Telephone: 800-233-0785
Fax: 614-466-9461
Website: www.ems.ohio.gov

Oklahoma
State Department of Health
EMS Division
1000 North East 10th, Room 1104
Oklahoma City, OK 73117
Telephone: 405-271-4027
Fax: 405-271-4240
Website: www.ok.gov/health/Protective_Health
   /Emergency_Medical_Services/

Oregon
DHS, EMS and Trauma Systems
800 NE Oregon Street, Suite 465
Portland, OR 97232
Telephone: 971-673-0520
Fax: 971-673-0555
Website: public.health.oregon.gov/ProviderPartner
   Resources/EMSTraumaSystems/Pages/index.aspx

Pennsylvania
Pennsylvania Bureau of EMS
Health and Welfare Building
625 Forster Street, Room 606
Harrisburg, PA 17120
Telephone: 717-787-8740
Fax: 717-772-0910
Website: www.health.state.pa.us/ems

Rhode Island
Division of EMS, Rhode Island Department of Health
3 Capitol Hill, Room 105A
Providence, RI 02908-5097
Telephone: 401-222-5960
Fax: 401-222-1751
Website: www.health.ri.gov/programs/emergency
   medicalservices/

South Carolina
SC DHEC, Division of EMS and Trauma
2600 Bull Street
Columbia, SC 29201
Telephone: 803-545-4204
Fax: 803-545-4989
Website: www.scdhec.gov/Health/FHPF/EMS_
   TrainingProtocolsRequirements/

South Dakota
Emergency Medical Services
600 West Capitol Avenue
Pierre, SD 57501
Telephone: 605-773-4031
Fax: 605-773-5683
Website: dps.sd.gov/emergency_services/
   emergency_medical_services/default.aspx

Tennessee
Office of EMS
665 Mainstream Drive
Nashville, TN 37243
Telephone: 615-741-2584
Toll-Free Telephone: 800-778-4505
Fax: 615-741-4217
Website: www.tn.gov/health/topic/EMS-board

Texas

Bureau of Emergency Management
Texas Department of Health
P.O. Box 149347
Austin, TX 78714-9347
Telephone: 512-834-6700 (press option 2)
Fax: 512-834-6714
Website: www.dshs.state.tx.gov/emstraumasystems/

Utah

Bureau of Emergency Medical Services
Utah Department of Health
P.O. Box 142004
Salt Lake City, UT 84114-2004
Telephone: 801-273-6666
Toll-Free Telephone: 800-284-1131
Fax: 801-274-0738
Website: www.health.utah.gov/ems/

Vermont

Vermont Department of Health
108 Cherry Street
Burlington, VT 05402
Telephone: 800-244-0911
Fax: 802-863-7577
Website: www.healthvermont.gov/hc/ems/
    ems_index.aspx

Virginia

Virginia Department of Health
Office of Emergency Medical Services
1041 Technology Park Drive
Glen Allen, VA 23059-4500
Telephone: 800-523-6019
Fax: 804-371-3108
Website: www.vdh.virginia.gov/OEMS/index.htm

Washington

Washington Department of Health
Office of Emergency Medical Services and
    Trauma System
P.O. Box 47877
Olympia, WA 98504-7877
Telephone: 360-236-4700
Fax: 360-236-4818
Website: www.doh.wa.gov/hsqa/emstrauma/

West Virginia

Office of Emergency Medical Services
West Virginia Department of Health
350 Capitol Street, Room 425
Charleston WV 25301-3714
Telephone: 304-558-3956
Toll-Free Telephone: 888-747-8367
Fax 304-558-8379
Website: www.wvoems.org/

Wisconsin

Bureau of Local Public Health Practice and
    Emergency Medical Services
P.O. Box 2659
Madison, WI 53701-2659
Telephone: 608-266-1568
Fax: 608-261-6392
Website: www.dhs.wisconsin.gov/ems

Wyoming

Wyoming Department of Health
EMS Program
6101 Yellowstone Road, Suite 400
Cheyenne, WY 82002
Telephone: 307-777-7955
Toll-Free Telephone: 888-228-8996
Fax: 307-777-5639
Website: www.health.wyo.gov/sho/ems

WORKS CITED

Ambulance Technician Study. *ECG Rhythms.* Ambulance Technician Study. (2012). http://www.ambulancetechnicianstudy.co.uk/rhythms.html.

Anderson, Paula. 2004. *Rhythm of the Month: Atrial Fibrillation.* Richmond, IN: Reid Hospital & Health Care Services.

Burns, E. *ECG Library.* http://lifeinthefastlane.com/ecg-library/ (accessed October 30, 2012).

Cardionetics. "Ventricular Ectopic Beats." *Cardiology.* http://www.cardionetics.com/cardiology/ventricular-ectopic-beats.php (accessed October 19, 2012).

Conn, F. "Syncope—When Passing Out Might Mean Passing On." E-Newsletter. (December 5, 2004). http://www.gihealth.com/newsletter/previous/045.html.

Float Nurse. "ACLS review: Acute Coronary Syndromes Part 5." *Float Nurse.* (December 4, 2011). http://floatnurse-mike.blogspot.com/2011/12/acls-review-acute-coronary-syndromes_04.html.

Mauvila.com. "Figure 9-3 Ventricular fibrillation (coarse)." *Mauvila ECG Tutorial.* (2004). http://www.mauvila.com/ECG/ecg_ventricular.htm.

Medicine-On-Line.com. "Rhythm." *Medicine-On-Line.com.* http://www.medicine-on-line.com/html/ecg/e0001en_files/08.htm (accessed October 19, 2012).

Peck, R. (n.d.). Retrieved October 19, 2012, from Rickypeck.com: http://www.google.com/imgres?imgurl=http://www.finlay-online.com/albarranschoolofmedicine/ekg14.gif&imgrefurl=http://www.rickypeck.com/ji-ekg-sample-strips/&usg=__esbKMuIXSJAUdGJqI-H8AdWMmfQ=&h=246&w=399&sz=53&hl=en&start=1&zoom=1&tbnid=z3n04vWKQd-OzM:&tb

Smith, S. "Cardiac Arrest suddenly after blood loss, is it due to MI? Also, when the rhythm looks like torsade, it is usually not." *Dr. Smith's ECG Blog.* (July 5, 2010). http://hqmeded-ecg.blogspot.com/2010/07/cardiac-arrest-suddenly-after-blood.html.

Szulewski. A. "Acute Posterior MI." Analysis and Interpretation of the Electrocardiogram. http://meds.queensu.ca/courses/assets/modules/ts-ecg/acute_posterior_mi.html (accessed October 29, 2012).

Thompson, A. "Long QT Syndrome Part III." *Paramedicine 101.* (September 15, 2010). http://paramedicine101.blogspot.com/2009/09/long-qt-syndrome-part-iii.html.

WSUPharmacy2015. *EKG Pictures.* (April 3, 2012). http://quizlet.com/11161507/ekg-pictures-flash-cards/.

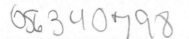

ADDITIONAL ONLINE PRACTICE

Using the codes below, you'll be able to log in and access additional online practice materials!

Your free online practice access codes are:
FVE6X46G0X33LGP3K71P
FVEW35IG3NUCV31208O5

Follow these simple steps to redeem your codes:

- Go to **www.learningexpresshub.com/affiliate** and have your access codes handy.

If you're a new user:

- Click the **New user? Register here** button and complete the registration form to create your account and access your products.
- Be sure to enter your unique access code only once. If you have multiple access codes, you can enter them all—just use a comma to separate each code.
- The next time you visit, simply click the **Returning user? Sign in** button and enter your username and password.
- Do not re-enter previously redeemed access codes. Any products you previously accessed are saved in the **My Account** section on the site. Entering a previously redeemed access code will result in an error message.

If you're a returning user:

- Click the **Returning user? Sign in** button, enter your username and password, and click **Sign In**.
- You will automatically be brought to the **My Account** page to access your products.
- Do not re-enter previously redeemed access codes. Any products you previously accessed are saved in the **My Account** section on the site. Entering a previously redeemed access code will result in an error message.

If you're a returning user with a new access code:

- Click the **Returning user? Sign in** button, enter your username, password, and new access code, and click **Sign In**.
- If you have multiple access codes, you can enter them all—just use a comma to separate each code.
- Do not re-enter previously redeemed access codes. Any products you previously accessed are saved in the **My Account** section on the site. Entering a previously redeemed access code will result in an error message.

If you have any questions, please contact Customer Support at Support@ebsco.com. All inquiries will be responded to within a 24-hour period during our normal business hours: 9:00 A.M.–5:00 P.M. Eastern Time. Thank you!